How to H—— ——————
Bones Faster. Bone
Fracture Healing Tips.

Learn About Bone Fracture Healing Foods, Types of Bone Fractures, and the Five Stages of Bone Healing.

By Dr. Ernesto Martinez

www.AttaBoyCowboy.com

Also by Dr. Ernesto Martinez

How to Travel the World and Live with No Regrets.
Learn How to Travel for Free, Find Cheap Places to Travel, and Discover Life-Changing Travel Destinations.

How to Boost Your Credit Score Range and Make Money with Credit Cards.
How to Repair Your Credit with Credit Repair Strategies.

How to Become Rich and Successful: Creative Ways to Make Money with a Side Hustle
How to Become a Millionaire: Learn the Best Passive Income Ideas

How to Heal Broken Bones Faster. Bone Fracture Healing Tips.
Learn About Bone Fracture Healing Foods, Types of Bone Fractures, and the Five Stages of Bone Healing.

How to Become Rich and Successful. The Secret of Success and the Habits of Successful People.
Entrepreneurship and Developing Entrepreneur Characteristics

How to Lose Weight Without Dieting or Exercise.
Over 250 Ways.
Learn About Foods that Burn Fat, Weight Loss Diets, Weight Loss Tips, Weight Loss Foods, and How to Lose Belly Fat

Cracking the Vitamin Code
How to Build your Own Supplement Stack. The Secret of Stacking Supplements for Beginners, How to Buy Vitamins and Minerals, and the Benefits of Dietary Supplements.

The Hardcore Program
How to build world-class habits and routines. Proven strategies for weight loss, success, and optimal health. How to form yourself into a new you through ritual and routine optimization.

How to Heal Broken Bones Faster. Bone Fracture Healing Tips.

Learn About Bone Fracture Healing Foods, Types of Bone Fractures, and the Five Stages of Bone Healing.

DEDICATION

T o all the friends, family, and healers that put Humpty Dumpty back together. Thank you!!

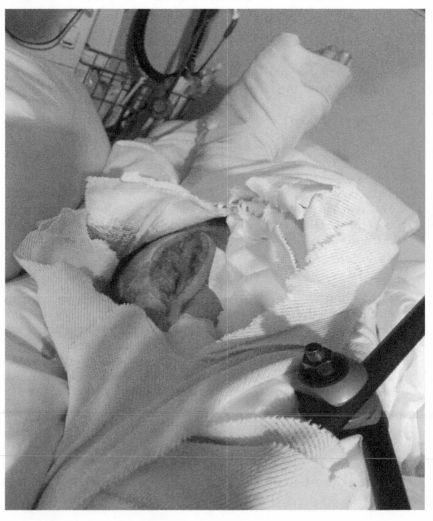

The broken bones resulted in the need for a fasciotomy, where the tissue around the affected area is cut open to relieve pressure and swelling. An additional surgery called open reduction and internal fixation (ORIF) was also used to drill metal rods into the bone to stabilize and heal the broken bones.

Table of Contents

Ernesto Martinez

Introduction

My experience with healing bones started at five years old when I stuck my right arm into an electric clothing wringer. It broke bones in my fingers and continued to break bones along my arm until my shoulder stopped it from progressing further. My babysitter had stepped out to talk to the neighbor while my parents were on the second floor taking showers so my yelling fell on deaf ears. My dad found me about an hour later and was so panicked he got an ax and broke the machine apart to get me out of it. It was the 1970s, and the ER doctor said it would be safer to just cut the arm off due to the extent of the nerve, muscle, and bone damage to the arm. My mom was distraught and immediately called my grandfather, who was operating a gynecology office in Ensenada, Mexico. He instructed my mom not to do anything and to wait for him. He drove 3 hours to Los Angeles and started treatment on my arm that same day.

My grandfather was a medical doctor who had a fascinating background as a trained naturopathic doctor, and thanks to his treatments, I had a fully functional arm cured without a single surgery. All that remains of that day are some extensive scarring caused by the synthetic fibers of my sweater melting into my skin.

After 30 years of practicing various forms of martial arts such as Kenpo karate, Seido karate, Jiu-Jitsu, Aikido, Judo, Shotokan Karate, Capoeira, and activities such as Greco Roman and freestyle wrestling, ballet, salsa dancing, basketball, cross country running, marathoning, baseball, football, swimming, and track and field focusing on pole vaulting, competing in sports has taught me that sports and exercise can hurt you. I've dislocated my left ankle by slipping on a wet basketball court caused by a leaky roof while competing in a basketball league tournament, I've torn the ACL in my left knee while playing basketball with college football and basketball players at the University of Southern California (USC), and broken my left clavicle and dislocated my left shoulder when my practical jokester wrestling teammate, Dong Kuo, body splashed me with his 274 lbs. body while I was wrestling someone else during practice. I've also cracked my sternum on three occasions, and broken my ribs eight times while playing football, basketball, and wrestling. I've even broken my knuckle on my left index finger after a fight broke out during a basketball game.

Lastly, my left lower leg shattered into more than 30 pieces after being assaulted by two guys and pushed down a flight of cement stairs. This last incident was the straw that broke the proverbial camel's back. Due to the extensive damage to my leg, the doctor recommended I amputate my leg or possibly face a fatal outcome.

I wasn't in agreement with having my leg amputated, so I contacted the top seven orthopedic surgeons in Los Angeles for a second opinion. One by one, each one turned me down and said it would be best for me to amputate the leg. After 20 years of helping other people heal their bones, it was time for me to do the same for myself on a larger scale. I scoured medical journals for broken bone cases, especially those from the USA Olympic team as they tend to have a lot of broken bones. The US winter Olympic team had the best information available. Using their data, my 15 years of schooling, my 20 years of practice as a clinician, and my personal experience with broken bones, I formulated a plan to get back on my feet as soon as possible.

Aside from the strong possibility of having my leg amputated and living a life with a disability, I faced some real existential threats such as bankruptcy, losing my home, and my life. Everything I had worked for was on the line. I needed to focus all my time, energy, experience, knowledge, training, and resources on developing a treatment plan to heal my bones or have my leg amputated.

The priority was to find a doctor that would operate on my leg. Luckily, I found a young physician named Dr. Saluta, who was willing to take on my case. He said, "I'll try, but I don't think it will work, and if it doesn't, we can just amputate your leg." My response was, "Absolutely not. I will agree only to repairing my leg. No amputations." He, thankfully, agreed. After the surgery, he said I would be non-weight bearing in bed for six months and in a wheelchair for two years after that, and that was only if the surgery was successful.

Again, failure was not an option for me, and neither was being in a wheelchair for two years. In the end, I was in bed for three months non-weight bearing, three months in a wheelchair, and three months on crutches. I went back to work in 9 months instead of the projected 2.5 years.

My healing started with studying everything I could about the science of bones. It took some time, but I firmly believe that the amount of time you invest in your healing is going to dictate your outcomes. I, like most people, did not have the time to wait two years to heal. I needed to get back to work or I was going to go bankrupt.

Coincidentally, while I was going through my recovery and rebuilding process, Kobe Bryant, the professional basketball player from the Los Angeles Lakers, was trying to recover from a tibial plateau fracture, the same injury I sustained. My injury, however, was much more extensive because my tibia shattered into 30 pieces, and I shattered the fibula as well. I kept track of how Kobe was progressing and noted he also struggled to recover. In fact, the injury ended up causing his early retirement. Unlike my other bone injuries, I was able to see and understand the magnitude of what this type of injury could do to someone. Kobe Bryant had unlimited resources, and I'm sure he sought the best available advice on every level. Given that he is a world-class competitor, I knew he had the right mindset and would not take any shortcuts.

My interest in Kobe Bryant led me to study other professional athletes and the issues they encountered while dealing with stress fractures due to overuse. This allowed me to learn from their successes and challenges.

How to Heal Broken Bones Faster. Bone Fracture Healing Tips.

Chapter 1: Human Skeleton and Bones

T he human skeleton is the building block and the framework of the body. At birth, we have approximately 270 bones. Due to some bones being fused at birth, some people will have varying amounts of bones. By adulthood, the total number of bones drops to 206 as more bones are fused as part of the maturation process.

Human bones are categorized into two groups: the axial skeleton, which contains the bones along the long axis or core of the body (i.e., the head and the torso,) and the appendicular skeleton, which includes the bones of the appendages. Since your body has two symmetrical sides, we have 172 of the 206 human bones as part of a pair including all 126 bones of the appendicular skeleton and 46 of the 80 bones in the axial skeleton. The 34 unpaired bones are bones along the center of the body which includes six skull bones, 26 vertebrae, the sternum of the chest, and the hyoid bone under the chin.

Bones make up the skeletal system, which also includes ligaments, cartilage, tendons, and joints. The skeletal system gives your body it's shape and works as a bony armor to protect your vital organs, including your brain, spinal cord, lungs, and heart. Bone is also a storage area for minerals abone brothnd vitamins, bone marrow, and fat. Your skeletal system also allows for movement by providing attachment and anchor points for muscles.

How to Heal Broken Bones Faster. Bone Fracture Healing Tips.

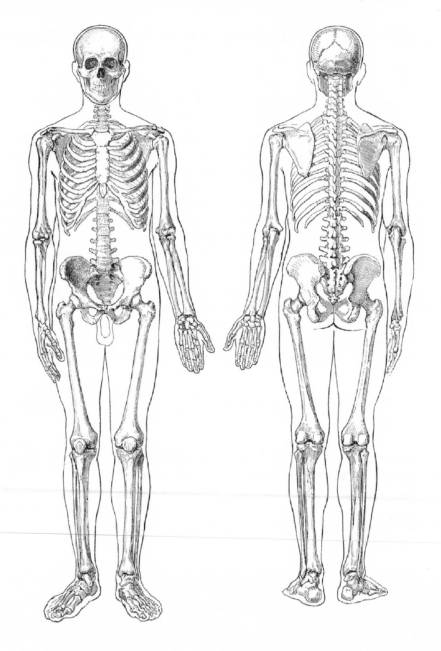

Structure of Bone

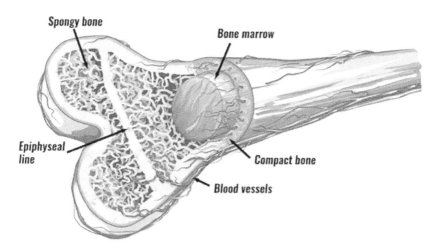

Spongy bone

Bone marrow

Epiphyseal line

Compact bone

Blood vessels

Bones are made up of two types of bone tissues. The first is compact bone, which is the hard, solid, and outside part of the bone. It is powerful and looks ivory colored. It has blood vessels and nerves running through holes and channels. The second is the cancellous bone, which fills the inside of the compact bone and looks like a sponge. The cancellous is where the bone marrow is found, stuffed inside of a mesh-like network of tiny pieces of bone called trabeculae.

There are two types of bone marrow; red bone marrow which helps produce blood cells and yellow bone marrow that helps store fat. As we age, yellow bone marrow replaces red bone marrow. Red bone marrow is responsible for hematopoiesis, also known as red blood cell production. The hematopoietic stem cells that are in the red bone marrow can develop into different blood cells, including platelets, which are used to clot blood and prevent uncontrolled bleeding, and red blood cells that work to carry oxygen-rich blood to the cells in the rest of the body. As the red blood cells age, they're broken down in the red bone marrow, liver, and spleen. Lastly, several types of white blood cells, which fight off infections for your body, are also found in the red bone marrow.

Chapter 2: How Bones Are Formed

A s you grow from a fetus, small islands of bone start to develop within the cartilage that makes up most of the skeleton. Osteoids build up in the cartilage and begin the process of ossification by depositing layer after layer of calcium and phosphate salts on the cartilage cells. Over time the cartilage cells die out and are replaced by cells called osteoblasts. Osteoblasts are responsible for the synthesis and mineralization of bone during both initial bone formation and later bone remodeling. Osteoblasts work in teams to build new bone called "osteoid" which is made of bone collagen and other proteins. As the osteoid is laid down, inorganic salts are deposited in it to form hardened mineralized bone.

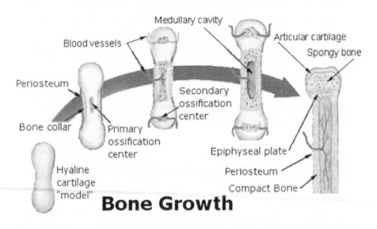

Bone Growth

The process of converting cartilage into bone is called ossification. Two types of ossification begin during fetal development; intramembranous and endochondral ossification. Intramembranous ossification is bone formed from connective tissue such as mesenchyme tissue. It happens mostly in the flat bones of the skull, mandible, maxilla, and clavicles. The four steps include; the development of the ossification center, calcification, trabeculae formation, and the development of the periosteum.

Endochondral ossification is bone formed from cartilage. It happens in the long bones and every other bone in the body. The steps are the development of a cartilage model, its growth and development, development of the primary and secondary ossification centers, and the formation of articular cartilage and the epiphyseal plates.

Endochondral ossification is how the majority of bone is formed and starts during fetal development with points in the cartilage called "primary ossification centers." These centers form the diaphysis of long bones, short bones, and certain parts of irregular bones. After birth, secondary ossification begins and forms the epiphysis of long bones and the extremities of irregular and flat bones. The epiphyseal plate, which is a growing zone of cartilage (growth plate) separates the diaphysis and epiphysis of a long bone. By 18-25 years of age, the skeleton will be fully formed, and all of the cartilage is replaced by bone, fusing both epiphysis and diaphysis (epiphyseal closure). In the upper extremities, only the diaphyses of the long bones and scapula are ossified. Cartilage remains in the epiphysis, carpal bones, coracoid process, medial border of the scapula, and acromion.

Chapter 3: How Often Bones Are Rebuilt

T he cells in your body aren't the same ones you were born with. The body is continuously breaking down old cells and replacing them with new ones. On average, every cell in your body is replaced every seven years. This is an average as some cells are replaced daily and some, like bones, can take as long as 25-50 years to be completely replaced.

Fortunately, the osteoclasts on bones can turn over in as little as two weeks when necessary, which allows you to heal bones with only a cast.

Chapter 4: What Bones Are Made Of

R einforced concrete is modeled after bone structure. The building structure is outlined with rebar, and concrete is poured around that to give it strength. The rebar provides concrete flexibility, and by preventing cracking, it makes the concrete much stronger and longer-lasting. Bone, however, is living, growing tissue. The bone structure is outlined with collagen a protein that provides a soft framework also known as the matrix (like rebar) and hardened with calcium phosphate, a mineral that adds strength. This combination of collagen and calcium gives bone strength and flexibility to withstand stress.

Main Components of Bone

- 10% of adult bone mass is collagen protein.

- 65% of adult bone mass is hydroxyapatite. Hydroxyapatite is an insoluble salt made of calcium and phosphorus (a ratio of Ca:P of 5:3).

- 25% of adult bone mass comes from water.

- <1% of adult bone has trace amounts of minerals including; magnesium, zinc, silicon, sodium, and bicarbonate.

Aside from the bone's mechanical functions, bones also work as a mineral reservoir. Bone stores 99% of the body's calcium and 85% of the phosphorus. Your body adds and subtracts calcium as needed from your bone and releases it into or removes it from your bloodstream. By maintaining blood calcium levels within a narrow range, your body can maintain optimal muscle and nerve function.

Chapter 5: How Bones Break

Bones usually have no problem supporting your body weight as you participate in daily activities. Bones are made to be strong, yet flexible enough to absorb the light impact your body experiences during activities of daily living. Sometimes, a bone is put under more stress than it can handle, and it breaks. Doctors call broken bones, a fracture.

The most commonly broken bones in the body are the clavicle, arm, wrist, hip, and ankle. Bones in the shoulder area are more likely to be broken because we use our arms and hands the most when trying to break a fall. The clavicle, also known as the collarbone, located between your shoulder and the front of the neck, is the bone that is most likely to get broken. The clavicles absorb the shock when you outstretch your arm to break a fall.

There are three main types of fractures: impact fractures, stress fractures, and pathological fractures.

Impact Fractures

Impact fractures happen when a bone takes an unforeseen, hard hit that puts more stress on it than it can handle. These usually occur due to a sudden impact, which causes the bone to snap. I sustained this type of fracture when I was pushed off a flight of concrete stairs. As I landed the weight of my 210-pound body was too much for my left lower leg to support, so it shattered into 30 pieces. Most impact fractures are caused by falls, being hit by something or someone, during sports, or an accident.

Stress Fractures

Stress fractures are some of the most common sports injuries. They're a type of repetitive stress injury that occurs when too much pressure is placed on the same spot of a bone over long periods. The pressure from the small impacts weakens the bone until it begins to crack. These cracks start very small and get bigger and bigger if they are not given a chance to heal. Stress fractures result from an imbalance between the strength of the bone and the force exerted on it.

To get stronger and faster, an athlete may overwork their body by repeating the same exercise over and over to become better at it and to build larger muscles. When the body is tired, your muscles will no longer absorb the shock from the activity as they usually would. Instead, the shock goes straight to the bone causing stress fractures.

Activities such as track and field, or basketball, that require running and jumping increase the chances of causing a stress fracture in the legs or feet. The long thin bones on the top of the foot and the heel bone are most likely to fracture. Stress fractures can be painful but will heal on their own if rested for a few months. The tibia bone of our lower leg is the most common bone to fracture at 24%.

Any sport that requires repetitive movements, like pitching or rowing, can also cause stress fractures in the humerus located in the upper arm. There are two types of stress fractures:

1. Insufficiency fractures: caused by normal or physiologic stress on a weakened bone.

Risk factors for an insufficiency fracture are osteoporotic bone, menstrual disturbance, immobilization, chronic steroid treatment, endocrine pathologies, renal failure, rheumatoid arthritis, radiotherapy, and complex regional pain syndrome.

2. Fatigue fractures: caused by abnormal stress on a normal bone.

Risk factors for fatigue fractures are morphological bone abnormalities and static pathologies of the lower limb.

Injury Prevention

- Keep track of your training schedules with a log

- Impact activities should be limited

- Physical activity should be increased slowly by no more than 10%-15% per week

- Equipment should fit appropriately for training demands

- Training surfaces should be optimized to reduce the impact

- Eat a well-balanced diet

- Calories in should be balanced with calories out

This chart demonstrates the relationship between the location of the stress fracture and the sport practiced.

Lower Limb	Sports
Femur (Neck)	Long-distance running, jumping, ballet
Femur (Shaft)	Long-distance running
Patella	Running, hurdling
Tibial (Plateau)	Running
Tibial (Shaft)	Running, ballet
Fibula	Running, aerobic, ballet, race walking
Medial malleolus	Basketball, running
Calcaneus	Running, long-distance military marching, skydiving
Talus	Pole-vaulting

Tarsal navicular bone	Sprint, middle distance running, hurdling, long-jumping, triple jump, football
Metatarsal bones	Running, ballet, walking
Base of the 2nd metatarsal bone	Ballet
Base of the 5th metatarsal bone	Basketball, tennis, ballet
Hallux sesamoids	Running, ballet, basketball
Pelvis	Running, ballet

Stress fractures can affect the functional prognosis of the lower limb, depending on the risk of fracture. There are two types of fracture: low and high risk. The classification depends on the location of the break on the bone, the prognosis, the treatment, and the complexity. There is tension on one side of the bone and compression on the other. Bones are more resistant to a compressive force, so the break begins on the side that is being affected by tension.

1. Low-risk fractures will usually heal with rest, they have a better prognosis, shorter healing time, and fewer complications. They typically happen on the compression side of the bone.

2. High-risk fractures will need longer healing time and more treatments such as casting, and surgery. Overall, they will have more complications if not managed in time. They usually happen on the tension side of the bone.

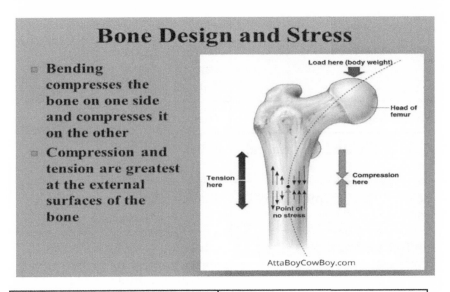

Bone Design and Stress

- Bending compresses the bone on one side and compresses it on the other
- Compression and tension are greatest at the external surfaces of the bone

Load here (body weight)

Head of femur

Tension here

Compression here

Point of no stress

AttaBoyCowBoy.com

Low-Risk Fractures of the Lower Limb	High-Risk Fractures of the Lower Limb
Tibia (postero-medial cortex)	Tibia (anterior cortex)
Fibula/Lateral malleolus	Medial malleolus
Femur (shaft)	Femur (neck)
Calcaneus	Tarsal navicular bone
Metatarsal bones (2nd to 4th shafts)	Talus
Pelvis	Base of the 2nd & 3rd metatarsal bones
	Base of the 5th metatarsal bone
	Patella (transversal form)
	Hallux sesamoids

How to Treat a Stress Fracture

If you suspect you have a bone fracture see your physician who will use magnetic resonance imaging (MRI) or X-ray imaging to produce a picture of the internal tissues, bones, and organs.

Treatment recommendations include;

- Stop the activity that is causing pain. Stress fractures happen because of repetitive stress, so it is important to avoid the activity that led to the fracture.

- Apply an ice pack to the injured area.

- Rest for 1 to 6 weeks. Once you can perform low-impact activities for extended periods without pain, you can start doing high-impact exercises.

- When you are lying down, raise your foot above the level of your heart.

- Take nonsteroidal anti-inflammatory medicines to help relieve pain and swelling.

- Use protective footwear to reduce stress on your foot or leg. This may be a stiff-soled shoe, wooden-soled sandals, or a removable short-leg fracture brace shoe.

- Your doctor may put a cast or fracture boot on your foot to keep the bones in a fixed position and to remove the stress on the leg.

- Use of crutches to keep the weight off your foot or leg until the bone heals may be required.

- Some stress fractures need surgery to heal properly. This is called internal fixation. Pins, screws, and/or plates can be used to hold the bones of the foot and ankle together during the healing process.

- If you have diabetes, see your doctor right away if you have pain or other problems with your legs, ankles, or toes.

- Slow pace

As you start to rehabilitate your stress fracture, you'll typically begin with one day on for activity and one day off. As you progress pain-free you'll slowly increase how often and how vigorously you exercise. If you resume the activity that caused the stress fracture too quickly, you can develop a larger stress fracture that will be harder to heal. If you re-injure the bone, you might end up with long-term problems, and the stress fracture might never heal properly.

The best exercises for a stress fracture are those that are non-weight bearing such as cycling and aquatic exercises. Switch to aerobic activities that place less stress on your foot and leg so that the stress fracture can heal properly.

Stress fractures take around 6-8 weeks to heal, so it's best to stop the activities that caused it. As long as you feel pain, the bone is still healing, and can break again in the same place. Consult your doctor before you do any physical activity on the injured foot or ankle.

Pathological Fractures

A pathologic fracture is a break in a bone that is caused by an underlying disease. Bones typically need a reason to break, like a trauma. However, some pathologies (diseases) weaken the bones. Forces, as slight as the weight of the body or a minor injury that would otherwise be tolerated, can cause a fracture in the diseased bone.

Some diseases like cancer or osteoporosis can make bones thinner and more fragile. These diseases make it more difficult for bones to absorb the nutrients they need to stay strong and flexible. They cause the bones to start breaking during regular everyday activities that would not usually cause a fracture in a healthy person.

Treatment of pathological fractures typically involves treating the underlying disease that is causing the break as well as the fracture itself. The success of the treatment often depends on the treatment of the underlying disease.

Types of Fractures

Fractures are further sub-classified by their complexity, location, and the shape of the break. The table below shows the common types of fractures. Some fractures can be described using more than one name, because it may have the features of more than one kind of broken bone. For example; open comminuted fracture.

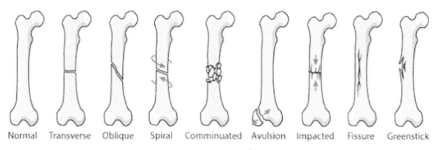

Normal Transverse Oblique Spiral Comminuated Avulsion Impacted Fissure Greenstick

Type of Fracture	Description
Transverse	Happens straight across the long axis of the bone
Oblique	Happens at an angle that is not 90 degrees
Spiral	The bone is twisted and pulled apart into segments.
Comminuted	Several breaks into small pieces between two large segments
Avulsion	In an avulsion fracture, the tendon or ligament pulls off a piece of the bone.
Impacted	As a result of compression one fragment is driven into the other

Fissure	Only the outer layer of the bone is broken.
Greenstick	Partial fracture in which one side of the bone is broken
Open (or compound)	At least one end of the broken bone tears through the skin
Closed (or simple)	Fracture where the skin remains intact

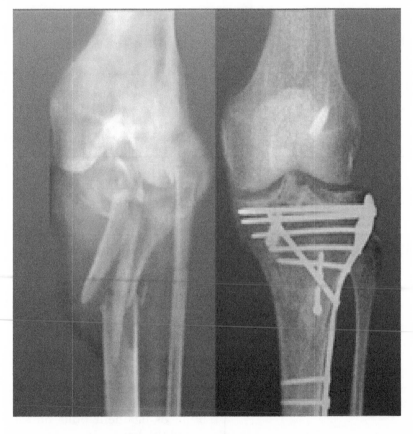

My Tibial plateau Fracture before (Left) and after (Right) was repaired with a combination of small metal plates, screws, and pins made of titanium or high-grade surgical stainless steel. Depending on the fracture type, the sizes can span 1.5 mm to 7.3mm. Screws inserted during surgical repairs do not set off metal detectors because they are non-magnetic.

Chapter 6: The Four Stages of Healing a Fractured Bone

1) Formation of Hematoma at The Break

When a bone breaks, blood flows from the vessels torn by the fracture. These blood vessels could be in the periosteum, osteons, and/or the medullary cavity. A blood clot forms in the area where the broken bone occurred. The blood begins to clot, and about six to eight hours after the fracture, the clotting blood has formed a fracture hematoma (Figure A). The hematoma contains a meshwork of proteins that provide a temporary plug to fill the gap created by the broken one. The disruption of blood flow to the bone results in the death of bone cells around the fracture.

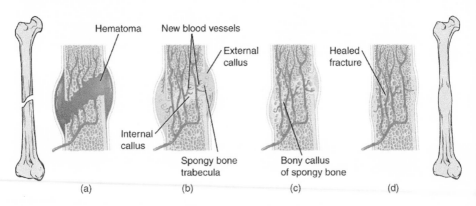

The immune system takes action and starts the inflammatory response, which is the first part of healing. Inflammation triggers stem cells from the surrounding tissues, bone marrow, and blood to migrate to the fracture. The cells start two vital processes: bone formation and cartilage formation.

2) The Formation of a Fibrocartilaginous Callus

Within 48 hours after the fracture, chondrocytes from the endosteum have created an internal callus (plural=

calli) by secreting a fibrocartilaginous matrix between the two ends of the broken bone. While the periosteal chondrocytes and osteoblasts form an external callus of hyaline cartilage and bone, around the outside of the break (Figure B), this stabilizes the broken bone.

3) Formation of a Bony Callus

Over the next few weeks, osteoclasts resorb the dead bone, osteogenic cells are activated, divide, and differentiate into osteoblasts. The cartilage in the calli is replaced by trabecular bone via endochondral ossification (Figure C).

4) Remodeling and Addition of Compact Bone.

After about six to twelve weeks, the internal and external calli unite, compact bone replaces spongy bone at the outer boundaries of the fracture, and healing is completed. A bulging may remain on the outer surface of the bone, but over time that area is remodeled (Figure D), and no external evidence of the fracture remains. The healing time, however, could be extended significantly If you have multiple breaks, ligament, tendon, or muscle damage.

Chapter 7: Cartilage

B one, muscle, and cartilage create the structure of our bodies. Muscles bend, stretch, and are flexible, while bones are rigid. Cartilage is between each of these other tissues. It is not as hard as bone, but less flexible than muscle.

Cartilage is the shock absorber of the body. It creates very little friction, due to the presence of synovial fluid that can be squeezed out when it is compressed or loaded with weight.

The primary function of cartilage is to hold bones together. It is mainly found in the joints of the rib cage, ear, nose, throat and between the bones of the back. Cartilage is a flexible connective tissue that resists stretching and is made of cells called chondrocytes.

Chondrocytes produce an extracellular matrix made of collagen, elastin, and proteoglycan fibers. There are no blood vessels in cartilage to supply the chondrocytes with nutrients. So, they get their nutrients via diffusion of nourishment from the synovial fluid, which fills the joint cavity. Because there are few nutrients available for repair, cartilage is not able to heal itself when damaged. Additionally, the chondrocytes do not replicate or repair themselves.

Three Types of Cartilage

Hyaline - the weakest and most common, found in the ribs, nose, larynx, trachea, and is a precursor of bone.

Fibro - the strongest type found in intervertebral discs, joint capsules, and ligaments. It is usually a transitional layer between hyaline cartilage and tendon or ligament.

Elastic - provides strength, elasticity, and maintains the shape of structure such as the external ear, epiglottis, and larynx.

Chapter 8: Factors That Affect Bone Healing

A pproximately 5-10% of bone fractures don't heal normally and are the result of delayed healing or non-union. Generally, the higher your bone mineral density (BMD) the faster your bones will heal.

Age: After 50 years of age your bone mineral density (BMD) starts to decrease, which makes it easier for your bones to break and prolong the healing time.

Sex: Men on average are heavier and have more muscle than women due to higher levels of testosterone. This correlates to a higher BMD for males, which makes it faster for males to heal bones.

Genetics: The heavier or taller you are the higher BMD you're likely to have. Because the bones have to be stronger to support the extra weight.

Race: Black people have the highest average BMD and Asians have the lowest average BMD. Whites and Hispanics are about average in BMD. Therefore, on average Asians tend to have the highest number of fractured bones and Blacks tend to have the lowest average of fractured bones.

Diet: Our skeletons are a product of what we eat or don't eat. The healthier you eat as a child the healthier your bones will be throughout life.

Endocrine system: Lack of, or imbalance of progesterone, estrogen, testosterone, growth hormone, growth factor 1, corticosteroids, or thyroid hormones can increase bone loss and increase the risk of fractures. Medications, exposure to environmental toxins (For example Phthalates and bisphenol A (BPA) found in plastics,) or exposure to endocrine disorders such as diabetes or hyperthyroidism, can cause osteoporosis due to hormone imbalances which damage bone growth and formation. Adequate control of blood sugar levels in people living with diabetes is essential because high glucose levels interfere with bone healing.

Physical Activity: The higher your level of activity the higher your BMD. The more you exercise, the bigger your muscles will be, and the higher your BMD will be to support the extra weight and torque from the pull created by those larger muscles. If you've sustained a fracture the amount of daily activity you engage in, and whether or not you're immobilized, will affect your healing time.

Lifestyle: During sleep, your body produces growth hormone and has increased bone repair activity. Therefore, sleep deprivation will impact your body's ability to build and repair bones.

Smoking will interfere and even prevent healing (nonunion) of fractured or surgically repaired bones. With less oxygen in your bloodstream, your body is going to struggle to keep enough readily available oxygen to keep up with bone, skin, and cartilage repair. This lack of oxygen will also increase pain levels.

Medications That Decrease Bone Density

- Steroids (corticosteroids and adrenal corticosteroids)

- Thyroid hormone

- Antacids with aluminum

- Chemotherapy

- Diuretics

- Anticonvulsants

- Phenytoin and Barbiturates

- Antibiotics

- Cholestyramine, cyclosporin A

- Gonadotropin-releasing hormone agonists and

antagonists

- Methotrexate

- Anticoagulants, including Heparin and Coumadin

- Lithium

- Benzodiazepines, including Valium, Librium, and Xanax

These medications can decrease calcium absorption which decreases bone density.

Factors for Low Bone Mineral Density That Can't be Changed

- Small frame

- Ethnicity

- Woman postmenopausal

- Man over 65

- Low levels of testosterone

- Family history of osteoporosis

- Long term use of corticosteroids, anticonvulsants, treatment for hypothyroidism, and chemotherapy

- Long term hypothyroidism

- Breastfeeding without taking calcium, vitamin D, or other nutrients

- Removal of ovaries or premature menopause

- Never had children

- Pregnancy without taking calcium, vitamin D, or other nutrients

- Breastfeeding without taking calcium, vitamin D, or

other nutrients

- Long term use of antacids containing aluminum

- Poor diet during childhood, adolescence, and or young adulthood

- Poor exercise habits during childhood, adolescence, and or young adulthood

- Former smokers

Factors that affect bone mineral density that can be changed

- Drinking more than 3 alcoholic beverages a week

- Smoking cigarettes

- Drinking more than one cup of a beverage with caffeine a day, especially the first two weeks post-surgery

- Not going out into the sun

- Drinking more than one soda a day

- Eating more than 12 oz of meat over a long period of time

- High protein diets for weight loss

Factors that can help

- Taking hormone replacement therapy

- Eating 3-5 servings of veggies a day

- Eating at least one cup of leafy green veggies a day in addition to the 3-5 servings of veggies

- Eating a balanced vegetarian or vegan diet

- Eating soy regularly

- Eating the recommended daily allowance of calcium

- Doing at least 30 minutes of weight-bearing exercise per day

Factors That Affect Peak Bone Mineral density

- Physical activity

- Hormones

- Risk factors

- Gender

- Genetics

- Calcium

- Nutrition

- Vitamin D; at least 20 minutes of sunshine a day will give you the vitamin D you need

- Peak bone mineral density is reached at age 18 for girls and 19-20 for boys and bone levels are static until the age of 30. After age 30 net bone loss starts to occur as bone resorption exceeds the amount of bone formed and slow bone loss starts.

- Being bedridden for an extended period of time causes excessive bone loss. Complete inactivity overtime doubles the amount of calcium excreted.

- If you're in bed for an extended period of time, taking 2000 mg of calcium a day will help replace the lost calcium

- Phosphorus in soda removes calcium from your bones.

- The more protein you eat the more calcium you excrete. Protein creates acid when broken down and the body uses calcium to buffer it.

- During Digestion, 1 ounce of meat requires 24 mg of calcium as a buffer.

- The older you get the more calcium coffee can leech from your bones.

- Smokers have double the risk of hip fractures.

Vegetarians

Most people eat about twice as much protein as they need. While vegetarians usually get the ideal amount of protein required. A plant-based diet is more abundant in nutrients than the average American diet and is generally lower in fat. Vegetarians have lower rates of many common health concerns, including osteoporosis, heart disease, cancer, particularly breast and colon cancers, high blood pressure, high cholesterol levels, stroke, arthritis, macular degeneration, and type 2 diabetes. Vegetarians are also usually closer to their ideal body weight.

During Roman times, gladiators were highly prized and valuable assets. These gladiators were trained, well-fed, and received good medical care. As part of their training, gladiators ate a mostly vegetarian diet and drank mineral-rich plant and bone ash solutions, after workouts for recovery and as a painkiller. This diet was believed to be the most effective at helping the warriors build muscle for strength during combat and increase bone mineral density for withstanding crushing blows from blunt force weapons.

During anthropological studies, spectroscopy was used to measure the stable isotope ratios of carbon, nitrogen, and sulfur in the collagen and the ratio of strontium to calcium in the bones. Physically the bones were found to have high bone densities and enlarged muscle markers on arm and leg bones. Similar to modern trained athletes, which is evidence of an extensive and continuous exercise program.

Plants contain higher levels of the metal strontium than animal tissues. Therefore, people who eat more plants and less meat will build up higher levels of strontium in their bones. On average, the gladiator's bones contained twice as much strontium as contemporary Ephesians bones. Historical reports show gladiators eating a diet of beans, barley, and dried fruits.

Regardless of the diet, you're following, make sure you increase your protein intake as bone reconstruction requires extra protein. Your calcium requirements will increase accordingly to the number of bones, and the amount of surface area that has to be healed. It's recommended to increase your protein intake 0.5 to 0.75 grams per pound of body weight.

Generally, a vegetarian diet will allow your body to rebuild your bones faster than a diet that includes animal meat. Animal protein creates a tug of war between digesting protein, and taking calcium from the body's reserves to buffer the acid being created for protein digestion. Consuming protein from plant-based sources lowers the need to deplete calcium reserves required to digest the protein.

If you include animal-based protein sources, use grass-fed, free-range, natural, hormone-free, chicken, eggs, pork, and beef or wild-caught fish. These types of meat are leaner, higher in key nutrients, including antioxidants, vitamins, lower in toxins, and have anti-inflammatory benefits.

High salt (sodium) intake increases calcium loss through the kidneys. Therefore, decreasing the availability of calcium for bones and increasing your chances of osteoporosis. Calcium dissolves easily into the bloodstream, and the increased rate of urination caused by high sodium intake will push more calcium through the kidneys into the urine. Reducing your sodium intake to 1 to 2 grams per day will help calcium retention. Avoid salty snacks and processed foods with added sodium, and decrease your overall dietary sodium intake.

Dairy products contain calcium, but also contain animal

proteins, lactose sugar, hormones, antibiotics, contaminants, and significant amounts of fat and cholesterol, in all but the low-fat versions. As a result, dairy products are not the ideal source of calcium.

Excessive amounts of protein in your diet will create unnecessary work for your body and create an acidic environment within your body. An overly acidic environment can cause demineralization (osteoporosis), muscle atrophy, fatigue, bad breath, and kidney stones.

Your body maintains a pH level between 7.35 to 7.45 to maintain homeostasis and for optimal functioning. Depending on health conditions, diet, or medications taken, your pH can increase and become more alkaline or drop and become more acidic. Not being in your optimal range can have negative health effects, so your body acts to maintain the 7.35 to 7.45 pH range. As the pH drops numerically your body becomes more acidic, and starts to take action to adjust your pH levels as needed. One of the strategies your body uses is to excrete calcium from your bones to neutralize the excess acid in your body. That calcium bonds with the acid and is excreted in your urine. The goal is to return your acid-base level to a healthy balance.

Chapter 9: Exercise and Fall Prevention

Falls

F alls are a big problem as the world population ages. Thirty percent of people over 65 years of age fall at least once a year, causing a negative feedback loop as those who have fallen are afraid to engage in activities for fear of falling, which causes further physical decline and causes more falls. Ninety percent of hip fractures happen due to falls, and up to 20% of people who sustain a hip fracture have a fatal outcome.

The incidence of falls increases with age as three sensory systems begin to decline. The vestibular system is the sensory system that provides a sense of balance and spatial orientation to coordinate movement with balance. It also tells you how fast and in which direction you're moving. The somatosensory system provides the body's position in space and detects movement. The visual system provides information regarding your body's position relative to the surrounding environment.

Exercises for fall prevention should be functional and focus on activities that challenge all three of these sensory systems. Activities such as walking on a ground-level balance bar, jump rope, or moving through an obstacle course, would test each of these areas at the same time and help prevent falls.

Whether it's osteoporosis or a patient who falls, exercising will help increase your bone density. Having increased bone density will make you less likely to fracture your bones if you fall, and if you do, it will heal faster.

Exercise

Physical activity or exercise can improve your health, reduce the risk of developing several diseases, and improve your quality of life. With all of the technological advances and conveniences we live with, it's more important than ever to start and maintain a lifelong exercise regime. Thirty minutes of exercise will cause a measurable increase in the production of energy-generating substances. The transport of energy between cells helps increase overall strength. Exercise increases energy and facilitates the removal of pollutants from the body.

Exercise causes your body to make more energy-generating mitochondria and causes the ones you already have to work more efficiently. Therefore, building muscle will increase your body's ability to create energy. Exercise trains muscles to burn more sugar calories and produce more enzymes that metabolize fat.

Exercise is even more vital during and after an injury to make sure your body recovers properly and maintains the gains from your rehabilitation. Research has clearly demonstrated that exercise is much more effective against depression than antidepressants. Almost any type of activity will yield health benefits, but two of the most efficient are weight training and swimming.

Weight Training

Stressing your bones with weight training will increase your bone density, reduce the risk of osteoporosis, increase endurance, increase strength, improve flexibility, improve balance, and can increase your metabolism to help you burn more calories for weight loss. Weight training also helps you remain independent and reduce or prevent cognitive decline as you age. Research shows that muscle builds faster when you increase load rather than repetition.

Swimming

Swimming offers unparalleled health benefits; it strengthens muscles, ligaments, and improves your cardiovascular fitness. Due to buoyancy, it provides a safe and effective workout, while gently supporting your body, particularly the injured areas.

Because water creates a thermal effect of sucking body heat away from your body, your body has to work much harder to maintain core body temperature. This causes you to burn a lot more calories than you normally would outside of water. Think about the times you've been swimming. Do you remember how hungry you felt afterward? That hunger was caused by the caloric deficit you formed while being in the water. If you hang out in room temperature water for an hour without swimming, you'll burn twice as many calories as if you had gone jogging for an hour. The colder the water, the more time you spend in the water, and the more activity you engage in water, the more calories you'll burn.

Swimming also puts less pressure on the body; the buoyancy of the water helps support your body weight, taking the pressure off joints. Depending on how much you immerse your body into the water will determine how much weight you put on your extremities.

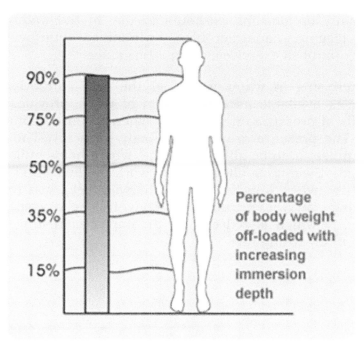

Percentage of body weight off-loaded with increasing immersion depth

The ability to grade the amount of weight off-loaded from joints makes swimming and other water-based activities the ideal option for people who have had lower extremity injuries.

Swimming is a non-weight-bearing activity, so you can still exercise in the pool when you are non-weight bearing. Just make sure your wounds are healed, and you have clearance from your medical team before going into the water. It can be a safe and comfortable exercise for people who otherwise might be very limited in their activities. Swimming is what helped me heal quickly and what I've observed as the most effective form of exercise for my patients.

Exercising in water also increases safety and decreases the risk of losing your balance, falling, and possibly hurting yourself if you were out of the water. Swimming is probably one of the safest exercise options for most people.

By varying your strokes and body position, you can get a comprehensive full-body workout while swimming. There are many options for workouts to use in the water from aqua jogging, aqua aerobics, swimming, aqua walking, water dumbbell exercises, or aquatic games.

Exercising in water is one of the best cardiovascular exercises available as every gallon of water provides 8.25 pounds of pressure on your body when you are submerged in it. The pressure around your body causes you to exert more pressure to be able to breathe, which helps build lung strength. Swimming allows you to work the heart and lungs at a time when injuries might otherwise keep you in bed. Exercising in water trains the body to use oxygen more efficiently which is reflected in an improved resting heart rate and breathing rate.

Chapter 10: First-aid Care for a Broken Bone

I f you suspect someone has a fractured bone, give first aid and get professional care as soon as possible.

1. If they're bleeding, stop the bleeding. Elevate and apply pressure to the wound using a sterile bandage, a clean cloth, or a clean piece of clothing. Do not apply a tourniquet. Doing so can cause the loss of a limb. If, however, you're unable to stop the bleeding and the person faces death due to blood loss, your only option will then be to apply a tourniquet as loss of life is more important than the loss of a limb.

2. Immobilize the injured area. Moving a broken bone can cause it to perforate blood vessels or nerves causing much more damage. If you suspect a broken bone in the neck or back, keep the person as still as possible to avoid permanent nerve damage or paralysis. If you suspect a broken bone in one of their limbs, immobilize the area using a splint or sling.

3. To control swelling and pain apply cold to the area. Wrap an ice pack in a piece of cloth and apply it to the injured area for up to 10 minutes at a time.

4. The person may go into shock. Keep them in a comfortable position, encourage them to rest, cover them with a blanket or clothing to keep them warm, and reassure them.

5. Call 911 or other professional help.

6. If the person doesn't appear to be breathing call 911 and begin CPR. As a precaution call 911 if: there's heavy bleeding, a suspected broken bone in the back, head, or neck, or a bone has punctured the skin. Otherwise, you can transport the person yourself to an emergency department by car or other means.

How to Heal Broken Bones Faster. Bone Fracture Healing Tips.

Chapter 11: Diagnosing a Broken Bone

B roken bones can resemble muscle pain or other kinds of injuries. The best way to confirm if you have a broken bone is to produce an image of it. This also helps the doctor determine how bad the fracture is and where it's located.

- X-ray is the most common way to diagnose a fracture. The X-ray image produces a picture of internal tissues, bones, and organs.

- Magnetic resonance imaging (MRI) is a procedure that produces detailed images. It is used for smaller fractures or stress fractures.

- A bone scan is a nuclear medicine test. The procedure uses a very small amount of a radioactive substance, called a tracer, that is injected into a vein, and scanned with a machine.

- Computed tomography scan (CT, or CAT scan): is a three-dimensional imaging procedure that combines X-rays and computer technology to produce slices, (cross-sectional images), horizontally and vertically, of the body.

Symptoms of a Fractured Bone

- Pain when the area is moved or pressure is applied.

- Swelling

- Bruising

- Skin discoloration around the affected area

- Angulation - the affected area may be deformed or at an unusual angle

- The patient is unable to put weight on the injured area

- The patient can't move the affected area

- Affected bone or joint may have a grating sensation
- Open fractures may be bleeding

Large bone (Pelvis or Femur) Fractures:

- The patient may look pale and clammy
- Dizziness
- Nausea.

Chapter 12: How Broken Bones Are Fixed

T he human body has its own process for repairing and reconstructing bone after an injury. Doctors help facilitate the process by helping provide ideal conditions for bone growth. The body then needs time to fix itself. After a fracture is healed, and in most cases, the area where the split occurred will be stronger than it was before the break.

PRICE

- Protection

- Rest

- Ice

- Compression (pressure)

- Elevation

Often a bone fracture may include soft-tissue injuries. PRICE is used to treat injured muscles, ligaments, and tendons.

Protection helps prevent further injury that could worsen the original one. Some strategies used include limiting the use of the injured area, not weight bearing on the injured body part, using crutches, and/or wearing a splint or cast.

Rest gives your body time to heal, prevents further injury, and increases healing.

Ice and compression can be used to decrease swelling and pain after an injury. Ice is enclosed in a towel or plastic bag and applied for 15 to 20 minutes at a time, as often as possible during the first 24 to 48 hours.

Compression is applied to the injury using an elastic bandage.

Elevating the injured limb helps reduce swelling by

draining away fluid. The injured limb should be elevated above the heart level for the first two days.

Depending on the type of injury, heat with a heating pad can be applied after 48 hours for 15 to 20 minutes at a time. Heat is used for pain management.

Reduction

If a bone has been dislodged from its normal position, it must be moved back (realigned, or reduced). Reduction is usually necessary if:

- Pieces of a broken bone are out of alignment.

- Pieces of a broken bone have become separated.

- Certain fractures in children do not need to be realigned because the bone, which is still growing, can correct itself.

Reduction is sometimes done without surgery (called closed reduction), by manipulating the bones or bone fragments back into place. After reduction is completed, doctors usually take x-rays to determine whether the fractured bones are back to their normal position.

More severe injuries must be realigned surgically (called open reduction). Reduction is usually painful, so people are typically given pain relievers, sedatives, or an anesthetic before the procedure.

After the bone is realigned, the injury must be kept from moving. Casts, splints, or slings are usually used after closed reduction of a fracture to immobilize the injury.

Traction

Traction uses weights, ropes, and pulleys to apply force to tissues surrounding a broken bone. During the early stages of healing, it is used to realign bone fractures, and hold it in the correct position. Traction is also used to ease the pain of a fracture while a patient is waiting for surgery.

Surgery

Sometimes your best option for repairing severely damaged bones is surgery. Surgery can help realign and maintain the position of bones when there are multiple broken pieces or a very complicated fracture. Open reduction and internal fixation (ORIF) is a procedure where hardware devices, such as pins, screws, rods, and plates, are used to align the bones in their regular positions or hold them together during the open reduction of a fracture. Sometimes these are temporary and will be removed once the bone heals, while other times, they're left in place permanently to support the bone.

Immobilization

Immobilization is another option after a fracture, it is used to reduce pain and helps heal by limiting the use of the tissue. During immobilization, the joints on both sides of the split are made immobile. Immobilization is used to treat moderate to severe fractures.

Occupational or physical therapists will outline a plan on how to maintain as much strength, range of motion, and function as possible during immobilization and how to improve them afterward. Immobilization is best used as little as possible as it can cause joint stiffness and muscle shortening (contractures), and muscle atrophy.

Types of immobilization used depend on the type of fracture sustained. Most fractures are immobilized with a cast, splint, or sling until they heal. Immobilization prevents the broken bones from moving, causing them to heal slower, and possibly not grow back together. If the broken bones have been separated or are out of alignment, they usually must be realigned (reduced) before being immobilized.

Splints

A splint can be used to immobilize some fractures, especially where immobilization is only needed for a few days. Splints allow you to apply ice to the injured area.

A splint can be prefabricated or made out of a long, narrow slab of plaster, fiberglass, or aluminum applied with elastic wrap or tape. The splint does not entirely encircle the limb, so it allows for expansion in case the injured area swells. Therefore, a splint does not increase the risk of developing compartment syndrome. Some injuries that eventually require a cast are first immobilized with a splint until the swelling decreases.

Slings are ideal for providing support and comfort for most shoulder and elbow fractures. The weight of the arm being pulled downward by gravity helps keep most shoulder fractures aligned. Slings can be useful to avoid some of the undesirable effects of immobilization. For example, if the shoulder is completely immobilized, the tissues around the joint can stiffen within days, preventing the shoulder from moving (frozen shoulder). Slings limit movement of the shoulder and elbow but allow movement of the hand. Aluminum splints lined with foam are used for finger fractures.

A swathe is a piece of cloth or a strap that is used with a sling to prevent the arm from swinging outward, especially during sleep. The swathe is wrapped around the back and over the injured part to hold the limb in place.

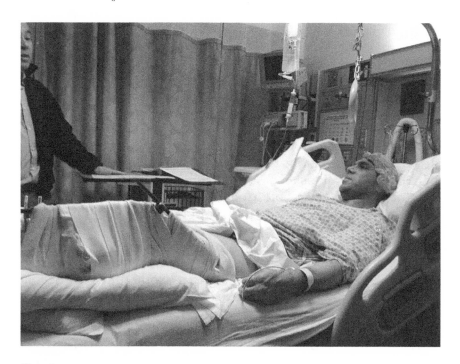

Cast

Casting and splinting is one of the most effective methods for facilitating bone repair. It protects the bone by immobilizing it to keep the bone in one place and prevents it from moving. A cast is a hard shell usually made of plaster or fiberglass and molded to the broken limb for comfort. A splint is rigid support, which is worn temporarily, and is easily removed. Tape can be used to hold fingers and small bones like toes together. Crutches are used to keep weight off from bones located in the leg or foot. In the upper extremities, a sling can be used in addition to a cast to hold the limb in place.

The cartilage in the calli has to stay in one place to be replaced by trabecular bone via endochondral ossification. The cast keeps the pieces aligned to prevent the bone from healing crooked. The cast provides support by taking the pressure off the break, so it heals faster.

If your child breaks a bone, a cast can help support and protect the injury as it heals, but a cast can't do its job without proper care.

Types of Casts

Plaster casts. Plaster casts are easier to mold than fiberglass casts and are generally less expensive.

Fiberglass casts. These plastic casts are lighter and more durable than plaster casts. It's also easier for X-rays to penetrate fiberglass casts than plaster casts which allows your doctor to give you updates on the healing progress without having to remove and reapply a new cast.

How to Reduce Swelling While Wearing a Cast

The application of a cast can sometimes cause a reaction in your body such as additional swelling. Swelling can cause the cast to feel tight and uncomfortable.

Three strategies to reduce swelling:

1. Elevate the affected area, for the first 24 to 72 hours after the cast is applied. Use pillows or cushions to raise the cast above the level of your heart. This allows gravity to assist with moving fluids out of the swollen area.

2. Apply ice to the affected area around the cast at the level of the injury. Place the ice in a plastic bag then wrap the bagged ice in a towel to insure that the cast remains dry.

3. Keep moving the affected limb by contracting and relaxing the muscles, and frequently moving the fingers or toes of the injured limb.

How to Scratch Under the Cast

A cast can cause the skin beneath to itch due to the build-up of sweat and dirt, the skin sloughing off, the healing at the surgical site, or even the cast itself rubbing against the skin. As you decrease the use and weight-bearing of a limb, the skin will begin to slough off and become thinner (making it more susceptible to tearing). To relieve itchy skin, point a hairdryer on a cool setting under the cast. Don't stick objects or use a coat hanger to scratch the skin. This can tear the skin, damage a surgical site, or cause infection.

Keep Your Cast Dry

Some types of casts might be ok to get wet, but generally you want to keep them dry. Allowing moisture to get between the cast and your skin can cause fungal infections, bad odor, or skin irritation. Moisture can also cause a bacterial infection at the healing surgical site.

If the cast gets wet use a hairdryer to dry the gauze and padding between the cast and the skin.

How to Maintain Your Cast in Good Condition

Remember that you're typically going to have the same cast for the next two months and it's essentially a piece of clothing. Keep the cast as clean as possible and if you're going to engage in activities that could get it dirty, wrap the cast in plastic to keep it clean. Avoid applying toiletries, powders, lotions, or deodorant on or near the cast. Leave adjustments to the therapist or doctor. Do not pull the padding out, trim, or break off edges.

Monitor Your Cast

Contact your therapist or doctor if the following occurs:

- Increasing pain and tightness
- Numbness or tingling
- Burning or stinging under the cast
- Development of excessive swelling below the cast
- Inability to move the toes or fingers of the injured limb,
- The limb becomes blue or cold
- The cast does not fit properly

- The presence of red or raw skin around the cast

- Cracks, soft spots, or foul odors in the cast

Chapter 13: How Cartilage is Fixed

C artilage, unlike bone, which can be set and reconstructs itself over time, is not able to heal itself when damaged. Cartilage is avascular, and because it lacks blood vessels, there are few nutrients available to be used for repair. Additionally, chondrocytes do not replicate or repair themselves.

Cartilage damage is difficult to treat, but there are some treatments available.

Arthroscopic debridement

For minor damage to cartilage, a cleanup procedure can be done to remove small pieces of damaged cartilage. During a washout, a small incision is made, and a video camera is inserted through the small hole and saline is sprayed to wash out any loose debris from the joint. Debridement involves cutting out damaged cartilage and is usually done at the same time as the washout.

Microfracture

For minor injuries smaller than two cubic centimeters, small holes are punctured into the hard surface between the bone and cartilage creating channels for the bone marrow cells to flow out and fill the crater. Blood clots rich in stem cells fill the holes and eventually remodels into fibrocartilage. This helps fill in the torn part of the cartilage and repairs the lesion.

Osteochondral Autograft Transplantation

Plugs of healthy tissue are harvested from an unaffected, non-weight bearing area of the patient's own joint. The plugs are installed in a damaged area.

Matrix-Induced Autologous Chondrocyte Implantation (MACI)

Cartilage cells are extracted from a healthy non-weight bearing area of the knee, then cultivated in a membrane for a few weeks. The cultivated cells are then installed into a damaged area of cartilage to help it regenerate.

Autologous Chondrocyte Implantation (ACI)

Similar to MACI, except that the cells are cloned in a laboratory for 6-8 weeks, instead of being harvested.

Stem Cell Therapy

Mesenchymal stem cells (MSC) are grown in a laboratory, then implanted in damaged cartilage to repair it. The MSC has the ability to differentiate into bone, cartilage, muscle, and adipose tissue to replace damaged cells.

Chapter 14: How to Prepare for Surgery

D epending on the type of surgery you're having done, you may end up unable to complete your business, work, personal, or activities of daily living for some time. To be able to focus on your healing, get organized. Make a list of things you need to get done and get them done before your surgery date. Follow your doctor's pre-surgery checklist and provided guidelines to help you be successful with your surgery.

Some items to consider:

Of course, we always hope for the best, but just in case, making a Will prepares your affairs so you don't leave your family with the burden of resolving your estate.

- Pay all of your bills and put future payments on autopay using online accounts.

- If you don't have the money to support yourself and pay your bills after your surgery then move or get a loan. You don't want to get evicted or have to struggle to keep your lights on while you're in bed recovering

- Depending on the type of surgery you get you may need help with housekeeping, grocery shopping, gardening, or running errands. Your options include using services such as TaskRabbit or TaKl for work around the house. Use Postmates, InstaCart, Uber eats, or your grocery store's delivery service to get your groceries. Another option would be to arrange to have a family member or friend help complete these tasks.

Adaptations for Your Home

You'll most likely have limited mobility after your surgery and find it difficult to move about your home. To prevent hurting yourself further, or putting yourself at risk for more injuries, you may need to make some changes in your home.

Home Adjustments

- Secure loose rugs with double-sided sticky tape around all edges, and remove area rugs, so they are not tripping hazards.

- If you have pets, consider boarding them temporarily so they are not a tripping hazard and so you don't have to repeatedly get up to clean up after them or feed them.

- If necessary, move your bed to the first floor or to a room that is closer to the restroom until your mobility improves.

- If your endurance will be compromised, then strategically place seats half or less of the distance between frequently traveled routes in your home. For example, if the bathroom is 20 feet from your bed and you're only able to walk 10 feet at a time, place a chair in the middle about 10 feet from your bed so you can take a rest if needed while on your way to the restroom. This will help you avoid walking longer than you can tolerate and increasing your risk of falling.

- If you have mobility, balance, or hip precautions then get handrails and/or raise the height of your bed to make it easier for you to get in and out of bed. Using cinder blocks is an easy and affordable way to raise the height of your bed. They are stable and strong enough to support the weight of a bed.

- High chairs, extra pillows placed on the seats, and chairs with armrests are recommended to avoid issues with balance, mobility, or to maintain hip or back precautions.

- Install temporary or permanent rails or ramps at the

entrance to your home for ease of entry. Items such as water hoses, loose doormats, or loose porch tiles should be removed to avoid a tripping hazard.

- In all areas indoors, and outside the home, remove anything that can be a tripping hazard such as stacks of clothes, books, magazines, extension cords, and children's toys.

- If you're in a wheelchair rearrange the furniture to clear a wide path through each room.

- Ensure entries and hallways are brightly lit. Add lighting and nightlights as needed everywhere you walk after dark.

- Keep a landline and a cell phone close by at all times.

Dressing

- Use elastic shoelaces, slip-on, or velcro shoes in case you can't bend over to tie your shoelaces.

- Use a shoe horn to help put on slip-on shoes. Avoid bending if you have hip or back precautions or compromised balance.

- A sock aid will help you slide on your socks without having to bend over.

- Use a button hook to help button shirts and pants if you have fine motor limitations.

- Zipper aids will help you zip up jackets, pants, or dresses. Again, great if you have fine motor limitations.

- Wear low-heeled shoes to prevent falls.

Kitchen

- Numerous adaptive utensils for eating and opening jars are available if you have fine motor restrictions.

- If you have jaw restrictions there are anti-spill sippy cups for drinking.

- Use built-up handles for eating or cooking utensils if your grasp is compromised

- Adaptive plates and bowls for eating help prevent food from falling out during mealtime.

- Stock up on water, juice, milk, or other drinks of your preference.

- Prepare food ahead of time and freeze it so it's readily available to be reheated when needed.

- Stock your pantry with easy to access healthy snacks that will help facilitate healing such as nuts, fruit, pudding, yogurt, low-fat frozen dinners, cut veggies, low sodium canned or instant soups, instant cereals, shredded cheese, pull-top tuna or other canned foods.

- Fresh food will speed your recovery, but if you have no other option stock up on healthy frozen foods.

- Stock pre-washed, pre-cut veggies and fruit to save time and energy.

- Save menus to local takeout places so food delivery to your home is easy.

- If you're on crutches, carrying food will be difficult for you. Consider small re-useable containers for milk, juice, or water you can slip in your pockets, so you do not have to carry a cup.

- If you'll be wearing a sling, consider buying pre-cut food or individual servings of food. Activities that require bilateral coordination will be limited so plan accordingly.

- If your surgery will affect one of your hands or arms, consider practicing daily tasks with your opposite hand before surgery. This will help you build up your non dominate hand/arm coordination since your bilateral coordination will be affected.

- Move utensils, pots, dishes, and small appliances onto the countertop within easy reach to save energy.

- Instead of lifting, slide pots and dishes along the countertop to save energy.

- To adhere to non-weight bearing precautions, and to conserve energy, sit while preparing meals. Use a seat that allows you to work comfortably on the surface you'll be working on.

Bathroom

- Install grab bars for the shower, tub, and toilet as needed to address decreased balance during showering or toileting.

- For hip or back surgeries add a raised toilet seat to make it easier to stand up and sit down on the toilet.

- If you anticipate having problems reaching behind during toileting, you'll need a long-handled toileting aid to help you wipe yourself after using the restroom.

- To help decrease fall risk, use bathroom floor mats with rubber backing and anti-slip shower and tub mats.

- If your balance is compromised or you have decreased weight-bearing, sit during showers. Use a shower chair, tub transfer bench, or combination commode for safety during bathing. To prevent falling, avoid bending over even when seated as you can slide off your seat.

- Use a long-handled sponge for reaching hard to reach areas, and to scrub your feet, lower legs, and back. This also prevents having to stand or bend over which can be a fall risk during showering.

- Use soap on a rope or soap in a dispenser so you don't have to bend over should you drop the soap.

- Use a detachable handheld showerhead during showers for hard to reach places and to save energy.

- Have a bedside commode in case you can't get into your restroom.

- If you have fine motor limitations use built-up handles for hair brushes, combs, toothbrushes, or razors.

- Use a waterproof cast cover for bathing.

One thing to keep in mind, and that often catches people by surprise, is that durable medical equipment (DME) are not typically covered by insurance. This meant that when I broke my leg, my insurance paid over $200,000 for my medical bills, but they would not pay for crutches ($200), wheelchair ($300), grab bars ($80), waterproof cast cover ($80), commode ($120), bone stimulator ($1200), circulating cold water therapy system ($150), or any of the other equipment that were basic necessities for survival once I left the hospital. It doesn't make sense, but that's the way it works and for most patients this added and unexpected expense leads them to avoid buying the equipment they need.

In my case, I was concerned about spending my savings and not having enough to survive while being off from work for 2.5 years while my leg healed. Some strategies you can try to get the equipment you need are: posting on social media a list of the DME you need. This has been a very effective strategy for myself and for my patients as there are lots of people who have DME from a previous injury. In my case my friend Octavio lent me his grandmother's extra commode, my friend Aharon lent me his mother's extra wheelchair, I rented the bone stimulator, bought the ice machine from craigslist for $20, bought other items on eBay, and made replacements for others. I used a plastic chair in the bathtub and shower, instead of buying a shower chair. Just be aware that the plastic chair is not as sturdy as a shower or bath chair and is not recommended for a heavier patient. I made a waterproof cast cover for bathing by wrapping my cast with a plastic bag and wrapping the ends with tape so water did not get in.

Chapter 15: How to Eat Before and After Surgery

Before surgery

There is a difference between eating to heal a broken bone and eating to heal after surgery. Healing a bone requires only giving the body what it needs to rebuild the bone, whereas healing after surgery requires supplying the body with the nutrients to support the immune system, prevent infection, as well as heal the bone, skin, and muscle. The caloric requirements post-surgery will be higher than eating to heal bone only.

In both cases, you're going to follow the same eating suggestions, except when surgery is recommended. Add increased amounts of garlic, onion, and citrus fruits (lemons, oranges, grapefruit, etc.) to your diet to help prevent infections and to promote faster tissue healing. Skin and muscle require higher amounts of vitamin C to heal than bone does. These foods also help boost the immune system to help your body fight off infections that could enter through the surgical site. Eat every 3-4 hours to avoid blood sugar swings and a drop in your energy levels.

Ninety percent of Americans think they eat healthy despite over seventy percent being obese. Disease-causing foods make up most of the standard American diet, with thirty percent of calories from animal products and over fifty percent from processed foods. Processed foods possess only ten percent of the original nutrient content of whole foods. Whole foods are also known as micronutrient foods, such as fruits, veggies, nuts, seeds, and legumes. Macronutrients are everything else.

Micronutrients fuel the immune system's proper functioning and enable the detoxification and cellular repair mechanisms that protect us from chronic diseases. The nutrient density of your diet will determine the nutrient density in your body's tissues. Studies show that focusing on food quality, such as eating nutrient-dense foods rather than calorie counting, is the easiest way to lose weight.

Dr. Mark Fuhrman developed this nutrient density scale to help people select a nutrient-dense diet and heal bones faster.

1000	KALE	119	GRAPES	34	SALMON
1000	COLLARD GREENS	119	POMEGRANATES	31	EGGS
1000	MUSTARD GREENS	118	CANTALOUPE	31	MILK, 1%
1000	WATERCRESS	109	ONIONS	30	WALNUTS
1000	SWISS CHARD	103	FLAX SEEDS	30	BANANAS
895	BOK CHOY	98	ORANGE	30	WHOLE WHEAT BREAD
707	SPINACH	98	EDAMAME	28	ALMONDS
604	ARUGULA	87	CUCUMBER	28	AVOCADO
510	ROMAINE	82	TOFU	28	BROWN RICE
490	BRUSSELS SPROUTS	74	SESAME SEEDS	28	WHITE POTATO
458	CARROTS	72	LENTILS	28	LOW FAT PLAIN YOGURT
434	CABBAGE	65	PEACHES	27	CASHEWS
340	BROCCOLI	64	SUNFLOWER SEEDS	24	CHICKEN BREAST
315	CAULIFLOWER	64	KIDNEY BEANS	21	GROUND BEEF, 85% LEAN
265	BELL PEPPERS	63	GREEN PEAS	20	FETA CHEESE
205	ASPARAGUS	55	CHERRIES	12	FRENCH FRIES
238	MUSHROOMS	54	PINEAPPLE	11	WHITE PASTA
186	TOMATO	53	APPLE	11	CHEDDAR CHEESE
182	STRAWBERRIES	53	MANGO	11	APPLE JUICE
181	SWEET POTATO	51	PEANUT BUTTER	10	OLIVE OIL
164	ZUCCHINI	45	CORN	9	WHITE BREAD
145	ARTICHOKE	37	PISTACHIO NUTS	9	VANILLA ICE CREAM
132	BLUEBERRIES	36	OATMEAL	7	CORN CHIPS
127	ICEBERG LETTUCE	36	SHRIMP	1	COLA

Pre-op Nutrition Guidelines

- Load up on healthy foods before your surgery, so your body has all the nutrients it needs to start rebuilding your body post-surgery.

- Eat lots of protein 0.5-0.75 grams per pound of body weight every day prior to your surgery. Protein will be essential for rebuilding muscle and bone post-surgery.

- Eating lots of fruits and vegetables is the best way to get essential vitamins and minerals for rebuilding your tissue. Green vegetables are great for skin, repairing muscles, bones, and cartilage because they contain loads of vitamins C, K, and magnesium. Eat a Traffic Light Diet Daily; a variety of green, yellow, and red fruits and vegetables.

- Whole grains give your body all the B vitamins it needs to combat stress.

- Reduce or eliminate sugars, caffeine, and alcohol from your diet. These create more stress on the body and actually remove nutrients from the body to metabolize properly.

After Surgery

After surgery, your body needs enough calories and nutrients to recover from the procedure successfully. What you eat can play a significant role in the length and success of your recovery, decreasing the risk of infection, and increasing your strength and energy. Avoid weight-loss dieting before and after surgery to ensure sufficient nutrients and energy for healing.

Pain medications can decrease your appetite after surgery. However, surgery increases the body's caloric needs to heal quickly, so keep track of the calories you're consuming to ensure that you're getting enough. Try eating smaller meals more often if your appetite has decreased. Another strategy is to drink meal replacement shakes. These nutrient-rich shakes are an excellent short-term supplement to meals after surgery.

Post-op Nutrition Guidelines

Here are some foods and nutrients you should focus on in your post-surgery diet:

- Due to the use of pain medications, a common

complaint after surgery is constipation. Fiber helps maintain normal bowel movements. At each meal eat fiber-rich foods such as fruits, vegetables, whole grains, and cooked beans. To prevent constipation, avoid dried or dehydrated foods, processed foods, dairy products, red meats, and sweets.

- Protein has essential amino acids that help with wound healing, tissue regeneration, strength, and building energy after surgery. Good protein sources include; eggs, nuts, beans, tofu, chicken, turkey, pork, seafood, and dairy. If you're having problems with constipation, avoid dairy. If you're not getting enough protein, add protein shakes to your diet.

- Fatigue is common after surgery, but eating carbohydrates can help restore your energy levels. Eating high-fiber foods like whole grains, fruits and veggies, and beans will boost energy levels and help prevent constipation.

- Healthy fats from olive oil, avocados, coconut oil, nuts, and seeds will increase energy levels, improve immune response and aid the body's absorption of vitamins.

- Vitamins and minerals are the most important nutrients in your post-surgery diet. Vitamin A prevents infections (found in orange and dark green veggies like carrots, sweet potatoes, kale, and spinach) and vitamin C helps the body heal wounds, prevent infections, and form bone (found in strawberries, citrus fruits, bell peppers, berries, potatoes, broccoli, tomatoes, spinach, melons, and collard greens.) Vitamin D (found in milk, fish, eggs, and fortified cereals) promotes bone health. Vitamin E (found in vegetable oils, nuts, beef liver, milk, and eggs) protects the body from free radicals. Vitamin K (found in green leafy veggies, fish, liver and vegetable oils) is necessary for blood clotting.

- Zinc to promote healing (found in meat, seafood,

dairy, and beans) and iron (found in meat and poultry, beans, apricots, eggs, whole grains, and iron-fortified cereals) are also helpful for wound healing and building energy following surgery.

- Ginger is an anti-inflammatory and helps with bone and joint pain.

- Gelatin has large amounts of collagen, which can be broken down into amino acids for rebuilding bone.

- Bone Broth contains important nutrients, especially minerals, that can be used in the bone reconstruction process.

Some foods should be avoided depending on the type of surgery and medications you may be taking.

In addition to eating foods that are rich in fiber, protein, healthy fats, carbohydrates, vitamins, and minerals, you must stay hydrated after surgery. Hydration is necessary for healing, absorbing medications, and removing toxins from the body following surgery. Drink at least 8-12 glasses of water every day after surgery to facilitate healing and stay hydrated. Bottled mineral water can be used to supplement mineral intake.

Water

Water is going to be one of the essential components of your treatment plan to help expedite healing. The amount of water you consume is going to affect how well and how long it takes for your bones to heal. Because bone cells are continually reproducing to strengthen and rebuild the bone structure, they require large amounts of water to facilitate the processes. Bones are not dry and brittle, but instead, contain up to 31% water and your body is made up of about 50% water.

Drinking eight glasses of water a day is the general recommendation. However, a more precise amount depends on your weight, activity level, and the environment where you live. For optimal health, drink between half an ounce to one ounce of water for each pound of body weight every day. For example, if you weigh 200 pounds, you should drink between 100-200 ounces (12.5-25 glasses) of water a day. If you exercise regularly or live in a hot climate, you're going to be on the higher end of that recommendation; if you live in colder weather and mostly sedentary, you'd need much less.

To assist with digestion and decrease hunger, drink one glass of water 30 minutes before a meal. Wait at least an hour after the meal to drink water to allow the body to absorb the nutrients.

Water brings nutrients to your bones, even if you eat all the recommended quantities, they will not make it into your bones without water. Water also helps move toxins and prescription medications out of your body. If you don't drink enough water, these substances can and do build up in the bones if there is not enough water to carry them away causing inflammation, breakdown of bone mass, and decreased bone density. If you don't meet the body's water requirements, it can cause several short-term and long-term health problems. Being dehydrated for an extended period can lead to several health problems like migraines, rheumatoid arthritis, angina, colitis, obesity, dyspepsia, hypertension, hemorrhoids, breast cancer, pulmonary tuberculosis, kidney stones, uterine cancers, and sinusitis.

When you wake up in the morning, you're most likely dehydrated because you've been without water for six to eight hours, and you lose water with every breath you take. Drink three to four glasses when you wake up every morning to rehydrate your body quickly. Add a dash of ocean salt or pink salt to help with balancing electrolytes and some fresh pressed lemon juice to make the water alkaline and lower your body's acidity. Many of the body's processes produce acid, which can lead to multiple health issues and slow your healing. Drinking lemon water will lower the acidity in your body and make you more alkaline. Having your body's pH in the optimal range helps facilitate healing.

The best water to drink is water that is not bottled or packaged. Water that has been packaged in plastic bottles is toxic as it contains residue and chemicals from plastic. One of them is phthalates, or phthalate esters, which are esters of phthalic acid. They are mainly added to plastics to increase their flexibility, transparency, durability, and longevity. The second most common is bisphenol A (BPA), an industrial chemical used to make plastics. Both substances have been found to cause several types of cancers, unbalance your endocrine system, and damage to fetuses. Your best option will be to use a reverse osmosis (RO) machine ($150) to filter your water. It can filter particles as small as 0.001 microns. The second, and much more economical option, is an activated carbon water filter, such as a Brita water filter ($12). Activated-carbon filters are rated by the size of the particles they can remove, and generally range from 50 microns (least effective) to 0.5 microns (most effective). Most toxic microplastics are about 2.5 micrometers in size. Either way, use refillable glass or metal containers to carry and drink your water from to avoid consuming some of these dangerous chemicals associated with plastic bottles.

Contaminants	Source	Health Hazards	Filter
Microplastics	Beverages in plastic bottles	Hormone disruptor, carcinogen	Carbon
Phthlates	Beverages in plastic bottles	Hormone disruptor, carcinogen	Reverse Osmosis
Bisphenol A (BPA)	Beverages in plastic bottles	Hormone disruptor, carcinogen	Reverse Osmosis
Atrazine	Herbicide used in agriculture	Hormone disruptor, carcinogen	Reverse Osmosis

Chlorine	Added to water supply in cities	carcinogen	Carbon
Microbes	Human or animal waste	Causes Gastrointestinal problems	Reverse Osmosis
Lead	Brass or alloy faucets	Hormone disruptor, carcinogen, neurotoxin	Carbon
Mercury	Batteries disposed near drinking water and industrial runoff	Hormone disruptor, carcinogen, neurotoxin	Carbon

Ten Benefits of Drinking Water First Thing in the Morning.

1. It helps you move your lower bowels for regularity in the mornings.

2. Water increases your level of alertness. It can have the same effect as coffee or tea, except that it won't cause further dehydration like coffee and tea due to their caffeine content.

Water will also stimulate faster growth of red blood cells in your system and generates more oxygen in your blood, which will boost your energy.

3. Boosts your brain capacity. Your brain is made up of over 70% water, and keeping it well hydrated will increase optimal brain activity. Not having enough water can cause fatigue, mood fluctuations, decreased memory, and reduced brain performance.

4. Strengthens your immune system.

5. Clears toxins produced during the nightly bodily repairs performed during sleep.

6. Boosts your metabolic rate for the rest of the day helping maintain an ideal body weight.

7. Promotes weight loss by helping you feel satiated, reducing your cravings for the day, and reducing overeating.

8. Releases toxins from your body, which improves skin complexion and radiance.

9. Water keeps your body hydrated, which is vital for the proper functioning of internal organs. Drinking water first thing in the morning prevents kidney stones and protects your colon and bladder from infections.

10. Staying hydrated will make your hair glow and keep your bones full of the water they need to grow correctly.

Signs You're Drinking too Much Water

Overhydrating is dangerous. It can lead to an imbalance of electrolytes in the body. If you consume too much water, there may not be enough of these electrolytes in your blood to keep your body working correctly. One sign that you're experiencing an electrolyte imbalance is swelling in the hands, feet, or lips.

A throbbing headache might be a sign that your brain is experiencing some swelling due to overhydration. Drinking too much water will lower your sodium concentration in your blood and can cause your brain to swell dangerously and possibly lead to irreversible brain damage, seizures, coma, or death.

When your muscles feel shaky or weak, drinking too much water can cause muscle weakness, spasms, or cramps. If your muscle pain or weakness continues even after you've reduced your water intake, it's worth checking in with a doctor. Drinking too much water can cause lingering fatigue.

When to Drink Water

- Drink four glasses of water immediately after waking, before brushing your teeth, and on an empty stomach.

- After your morning flush drink 12 ounces (1.5 cups) every two hours.

- Do not eat anything for the next 45 minutes.

- After 45 minutes, you may eat and drink as normal.

- Do not eat or drink anything for 2 hours after breakfast, lunch, and dinner.

Generally, it takes about a week to get accustomed to increased water intake. Just make sure you drink about the same amount every day.

Facilitate the creation of exclusion zone (EZ) water in your body

Dr. Pollack, Professor of Biochemical Engineering at the University of Washington, discovered EZ water, also known as structured water. EZ water is the water used by cells, and it's very different from drinking water. It is viscous like honey, somewhere between solid and liquid. EZ water is a particular type of water that forms in your cells. EZ water energizes your mitochondria, prevents aging, reduces stress, and speeds recovery. It's like a charged battery that can deliver energy to cells when needed. EZ water increases the mitochondria's ability to produce more power. It improves protein folding, the physical process by which a protein chain becomes biologically functional.

1. EZ water forms naturally in raw vegetable juice and spring water.
2. EZ water forms when you blend water or butterfat into the water for 30 seconds.

3. EZ water forms in your cells when you expose your skin and eyes to unfiltered sunlight for a few minutes every day without clothing, sunglasses, or sunscreen. The more skin you uncover, the more EZ water you'll make.

4 Stand on a vibration plate for up to 15 minutes.

5. Use Red light therapy to expose the body to red light, the longest wavelength of visible light on the visible light spectrum, through 1200 nm radiation, creating EZ water that spreads throughout your entire body.

6. Sitting in an infrared sauna will give you a concentrated dose of 1200 nm light and make lots of EZ water.

Chapter 16: Types of Weight-Bearing Status

W eight-bearing is the amount of weight a patient can put on an injured body part for optimal healing. When starting to weight bear, know the difference between good pain (muscle, nerve) and bad (bone, which indicates the bone is still broken). Check-in with your doctor, physical or occupational therapist, to understand your specific weight-bearing restrictions and how to maintain them properly.

It is essential to strictly adhere to your weight-bearing restrictions after surgery or injury, otherwise, you can disrupt healing and delay your recovery. These restrictions are meant to protect your body as it is healing.

If you fail to maintain your weight-bearing status appropriately, you could risk causing further injury or jeopardizing the success of your surgery.

Non-weight bearing (NWB): The bone is not permitted to support any weight at all. If the leg is non-weight bearing, the patient may hop on the other leg or use crutches, wheelchair, or other devices for mobility. In this example, 0% of the body weight may be rested on the leg.

Touch-down weight-bearing (TDWB) or Toe-touch weight-bearing (TTWB): The arm, foot, or toes may touch a surface to maintain balance, but is not to support any weight (0 to 20 percent of body weight). When touch down weight bearing, imagine having an egg under your foot and you want to avoid crushing it.

Partial weight-bearing (PWB): A small amount of weight may be supported by the affected limb (20 to 50 percent). This would allow for supporting body weight, but not the full body weight on the limb. This would permit you to stand with your body weight evenly supported by both feet, but not to walk. As full weight-bearing is still not allowed, crutches, a cane, or walker can help you walk without losing your balance.

Weight-bearing as tolerated: The person determines the amount of weight (50-100 percent) they can tolerate on the affected limb.

Full weight-bearing: The limb can carry 100 percent of the body weight, which allows for normal activity.

Symptoms that may indicate you need to see your doctor if you break your weight-bearing status may include:

- Increased pain in your injured or operated leg

- An increase in redness or swelling in your leg

- Difficulty moving around that causes more pain

- If you've broken weight-bearing precautions after an injury or surgery and you feel discomfort, it's best to contact your doctor and explain what has happened.

Chapter 17: Best Types of Exercise for Bone Repair

T he more weight your bones support during physical activity, the faster they're going to heal. This has to be balanced with the injury that was sustained. Follow your physician's directions as to your weight-bearing status, otherwise, you can cause additional fractures which can prolong the healing process. The higher your level of physical activity at any stage in life, the higher your bone mineral density will be. Physical activity also promotes increased oxygen circulation through your system which in turn speeds up healing.

Wolff's Law: The use it or lose it principle. When mechanical strain is put on your bones, this triggers osteoclasts, osteoblasts, and osteocytes to produce more bone to support the mechanical load on them. Repetitive loading of bone will cause an adaptive response with bone growth and remodeling in response to the forces that are placed upon it, enabling the bone to better cope with these loads.

With weight-bearing status in mind, you want to engage in targeted bone loading (TBL) during physical activity. TBL is a force-generating activity that targets a specific bone or region beyond that which is provided by typical activities of daily living. Physical activity is bodily movement beyond typical levels of exertion. Exercise is a planned repetitive, purposeful, and targeted activity. For example, gardening and shopping are physical activities, whereas swimming is an exercise and physical activity, but none of these activities are targeted bone loading. Although physical activity and exercise are both beneficial, TBL on a leg fracture, whose weight-bearing status has been upgraded to full weight-bearing, would target that specific limb for rehabilitation. Full weight-bearing means you can engage in normal activities as tolerated. Hopping or standing on one leg would be an example of targeting the specific bone for loading.

One of my favorite weight-bearing exercises is bouncing on a trampoline. It takes you from weightless to as much as four times G-Force in resistance with every bounce. NASA uses rebounding on trampolines to increase bone density in astronauts. The same benefits can be achieved by anyone trying to improve their bone density. Trampoline use also helps build your balance and core strength which helps reduce the incidence of falls in people who have decreased stability.

The more exercise or mechanical loading you do, the more your mesenchymal stem cells in your bone marrow will make osteoblasts which will form more bone. Exercises such as weight training will promote building stronger bones much faster than almost any other exercise. The less active you are, the more those cells will produce adipocyte fat cells instead.

Examples of Weight-Bearing Exercises:

- Walking

- Hiking

- Dancing

- Stair climbing

- Strength training: lifting weights and/or using exercise bands will increase bone density and decrease the chances of a fracture.

- Bodyweight exercises

- Flexibility exercises are good for joints and mobility and for avoiding fractures. Stretching, yoga, and tai chi are good for posture, balance, and strength.

No matter what type of bone fracture you have, some sort of physical exercise is necessary to speed the healing process. If you're non-weight bearing, that means you are non-weight bearing only on the affected area, and you can still engage in some type of exercise as recommended by your doctor or therapist. Lack of exercise or too much high-intensity exercise will cause bone loss. Too much training or high-intensity exercise causes bone loss.

If you've had surgery, exercising in water is ideal once your incisions are closed. Water allows you to exercise without placing your full weight on the affected limb. The water helps support part of your body weight, so you can simply grade your movement through the water and grade the amount of exertion you want to place on the muscles, joints, and bone. The water also cools your body and keeps you hydrated during activity. Although swimming has many benefits, it isn't weight-bearing, therefore its better at working your muscles than your bones.

Water exercise such as aqua jogging, aqua aerobics, or swimming is the gold standard for any recovery. The water offers constant hydration, unparalleled safety because you don't have to worry about falling, and the amount of weight you put on your joints and muscles can easily be graded. One of the major issues with exercise recovery and trauma is inflammation. Exercising and water help combat this major issue. It keeps your temperature down, and it does not allow for excess heat creation within the joints or the area that has been damaged.

The temperature differential between the water and your body also allows for thermal conduction which increases calorie burning, vasodilation, and vasoconstriction to help increase blood flow, oxygen, nutrients, and immune system response to the areas in need. It's kind of like putting your entire body on a healing fast track. It does, however, cause you to burn more calories which could be beneficial if you need to lose weight during this process. If you don't need to lose extra weight then you can offset the weight loss by consuming extra calories, which in turn can be beneficial in that it will give your healing bones more access to needed nutrients.

Examples of non-weight bearing exercises:

- Lifting weights or using resistance bands while seated.

- Swimming, water aerobics, or rowing.

- Using a hand bike to work your upper body.

- Riding a bicycle or using a stationary bicycle.

- Range of motion exercises for joint flexibility.

Exercise should be done at least 3 days a week for about an hour at a time. Use a program that you can stick to long term and adjust as needed. Don't go into extreme workout regimes for a few weeks then stop. That doesn't help you much.

Chapter 18: How to Sleep for Increased Bone Healing

I t's not the amount of sleep that will help you heal faster, but the quality of the sleep. Most people require between eight to ten hours of sleep a day. However, if you're feeling tired after surgery or exercise and feel like you need more sleep than usual, then sleep as much as your body is asking you for.

During sleep, your brain's immune cells produce a vital substance called interleukin 12, which is responsible for making you smarter, giving you energy, and building immunity to disease. This is the reason why you wake up in the morning feeling refreshed.

Sleep is vital to the release of human growth hormone (HGH). HGH is released by the brain into the bloodstream during deep sleep. Up to 75% of HGH is released during deep sleep and 25% during exercise. HGH is part of the repair and restoration function of the body. It is going to become even more important as your body is trying to heal from broken bones.

Because you may be experiencing pain from your fractured or surgically repaired bone, you may need pain or sleeping medication to help you sleep depending on the level of pain. Stay away from caffeine, nicotine, and alcohol which can all have a stimulating effect and disturb your sleep. The highest concentrations of HGH are released during slow-wave sleep (SWS) which starts a few hours after sleeping has started. Therefore, try to avoid naps after 3 pm, so that you're more tired at night and you'll sleep for prolonged periods of time.

Fifteen ways to Improve your sleep

1. Increase light exposure during the day. Your body has a natural time-keeping clock known as your circadian rhythm. It affects your brain, body, and hormones, helping

you stay awake and telling your body when it's time to sleep. Natural sunlight or bright light during the day helps keep your circadian rhythm healthy, Improves daytime energy, as well as nighttime sleep quality and duration.

2. Reduce blue light exposure in the evening. Exposure to light at night disrupts your circadian rhythm, tricking your brain into thinking it is still daytime. It reduces hormones like melatonin, which helps you relax and get deep sleep. Blue light, which electronic devices like smartphones and computers emit in large amounts, is the most disruptive.

3. Don't consume caffeine late in the day. When consumed late in the day, coffee stimulates your nervous system and may stop your body from naturally relaxing at night.

4. Try to sleep and wake at consistent times. Your body's circadian rhythm functions on a set loop, aligning itself with the sunrise and sunset. Being consistent with your sleep and waking times can aid long-term sleep quality

5. Take a melatonin supplement. Melatonin is an essential sleep hormone that tells your brain when it's time to relax and head to bed. Melatonin may be one of the easiest ways to fall asleep.

6. Other sleep supplements;

- Ginkgo biloba: A natural herb with many benefits, it may aid in sleep, relaxation, and stress reduction, but the evidence is limited. Take 250 mg 30–60 minutes before bed.

- Glycine: A few studies show that 3 grams of the amino acid glycine can improve sleep quality

- Valerian root: Several studies suggest that valerian can help you fall asleep and enhance the quality of sleep. Take 500 mg before bed.

- Magnesium: Responsible for over 600 reactions within your body, magnesium can improve relaxation and enhance sleep quality

- L-theanine: An amino acid, l-theanine, can promote relaxation and sleep. Take 100–200 mg before bed.

- Lavender: A powerful herb with many health benefits, lavender can induce a calming and sedentary effect to improve sleep. Take 80–160 mg containing 25–46% linalool.

7. Drinking alcohol at night can negatively affect your sleep and hormones. Alcohol is known to cause or increase the symptoms of sleep apnea, snoring, and disrupted sleep patterns.

8. Optimize your bedroom environment. To optimize your bedroom environment, try to minimize external noise, uncomfortable temperatures, bright light, and artificial lights from devices like alarm clocks. Make sure your bedroom is a quiet, relaxing, clean, and enjoyable place.

9. Late-night eating will negatively impact sleep quality and the natural release of HGH and melatonin.

10. Relax and clear your mind in the evening. Strategies include listening to relaxing music, reading a book, meditating, deep breathing, and visualization.

11. A relaxing bath or shower is another popular way to sleep better.

12. Get a comfortable bed, mattress, and pillow.

13. Although daily exercise is critical for a good night's sleep, performing it too late in the day may cause sleep problems.

14. Drinking liquids before bed can cause excessive urination during the night affecting sleep quality and daytime energy.

15. Wear loose cotton clothing or go bare. Remove anything that would limit circulation such as a bra, elastic underwear, socks, or jewelry. If you're prescribed a brace or splint for your injury, ask if they are to be worn at night or

only during activity. Only use your splints or braces as prescribed. Wearing them more than is necessary can reduce circulation and further decrease strength. Reduced blood flow can translate to reduced healing and increased work for your body.

Chapter 19: Caloric Intake to Facilitate Bone Healing

To repair damaged bone, your body is going to require more calories than usual to reconstruct the damaged bone. Exactly how much depends on your age, health, metabolic rate, level of conditioning, and the extent of your bone fracture. As a general rule, your body is going to need 15-20% more calories than usual.

When I broke my leg, I was training for a wrestling meet and was exercising twice a day. I was in excellent physical condition, I ate mostly organic, and vegetarian. Before the accident I weighed 210 pounds and had low body fat at 14%, within a few weeks after my surgeries I weighed 170 pounds. Even though I was mostly in bed, I felt hungry all the time and my food intake increased by about 50%. Even with the increase in consumption, I was losing weight, and could not eat enough to keep my weight up. I tried several strategies and I started eating foods that were higher in calories like whole milk kefirs, creamed spinach, and swiss cheese. I ended up doubling my normal caloric intake, just to maintain and boost my weight slightly to 180 pounds.

Once I got my weight up to 180 pounds, I could feel fat coming on, so I started cutting the calories back down to around 150% of my normal caloric intake. The point is you have to keep track of your weight and adjust your eating habits accordingly. If you're overweight, to begin with, then losing some weight is a good idea. It'll make your rehabilitation easier and faster. However, this is not the time to diet. Your body is going to need a variety of nutrients that need to be eaten daily to help speed up recovery.

As I healed and my body stopped needing the high caloric intake, the insatiable hunger I had been feeling started to disappear. This led me to stop craving the high-calorie foods I had been eating and to start eating much less at mealtimes.

Chapter 20: How to Eat for Rapid Bone Healing

O ver the years I have studied dozens of eating plans, and I believe the Zone Diet is the most practical even though the name is misleading because the word "diet" seems restrictive. This diet helps you eat foods during mealtime in the right proportions: 40 percent carbs, 30 percent protein, and 30 percent fat. This helps keep your insulin and other inflammation-promoting hormones "in the zone," not too high or low which keeps your body in ideal conditions for healing.

Before my accident, and after I was healed, I practiced intermittent fasting eating within a four-hour window each day. Usually between 12-4 pm. However, during the healing process, I found it to be impractical to help facilitate faster healing. Aside from forming a baby, building bone is the second most energy-intensive activity the body has to engage in. During bone rebuilding, your body is going to be doing extra work 24 hours a day. Your body will take what nutrients it needs from the foods you eat. Some of the nutrients will be stored and what the body doesn't need will be discharged. For instance, when you eat a salad, your body will absorb the vitamin C that it needs, but because the body doesn't store extra vitamin C, any additional vitamin C eaten during the meal will be discharged. Vitamin C, however, is vital to rebuilding body tissue and your body will need more than usual. If your next meal is lacking vitamin C, your body's healing process will be slowed due to the lack of nutrients. This scenario can repeat itself for other vital nutrients as well.

To ensure a steady supply of needed nutrients to heal bone faster, it is recommended to eat a small meal every two hours.

Sample Meal Plan

Breakfast
Omelet with spinach, onion, feta cheese, avocado, and

cooked in coconut oil.

Fruit salad with pineapple, guava, strawberries, chia seeds, and walnuts

Slice of Ezekiel Bread with almond butter

Lunch

Salad made with parsley, mixed lettuce greens, broccoli, chickpeas, kidney beans, peas, soybeans, blue cheese, and olive oil.

Glass of green tea

Snack

Trail mix, orange, cup of kefir

Dinner

Soy meat or organic animal protein source, buckwheat, and seaweed.

Carrot and pineapple salad for dessert.

Snack

Healthy bone and joint shake

Healthy Bone and Joint Shake

Use a Vitamix 64-ounce blender to blend the ingredients below and refrigerate in glass bottles.
- 1/2 cup of Vegan protein powder or three large pastured eggs or homemade protein powder (see recipe below)
- 1 teaspoon turmeric
- 1 teaspoon Ceylon cinnamon
- 1 teaspoon cocoa powder
- 2 tablespoons of chopped raw ginger
- 1 teaspoon of flaxseed oil
- 1 teaspoon of bee pollen
- 1 teaspoon of royal jelly

- 1 teaspoon of pure vanilla extract
- 1 tablespoon of Brazil nuts
- 1 tablespoon of almonds
- 1 tablespoon of pumpkin seeds
- 1 cup of mixed berries (blueberries, raspberries, and/or blackberries).
- 1 cup of mixed greens (baby spinach, swiss chard, and/or arugula)
- Optional flavor with raw honey or stevia as needed

Fill to the top with water, bone broth, or if you prefer a creamy texture use almond or oat milk.

Homemade Protein Powder

Avoid commercial protein powders, most are high in toxic metals such as arsenic, cadmium, lead, and mercury. Many also contain added oils, artificial sweeteners, bisphenol-A (BPA, used to make plastic), pesticides, or other contaminants with links to cancer and other health conditions. High doses can cause increased bowel movements, nausea, dehydration, bloating, cramps, reduced appetite, fatigue, and headache.

Protein shakes are meant to supplement your diet occasionally and not to be used daily or replace whole foods. If you're going to use protein shakes, consider making your own.

To make your protein powder, start with a protein base. Commercial protein powders are made with dairy, so if you prefer something similar, use dry milk or whey. For plant-based protein, you can use whole nuts or seeds, such as almonds, sunflower seeds, or pumpkin seeds. Protein-rich flours like buckwheat, quinoa, chickpea, or yellow pea are also a good option. Mix ½ cup of the protein powder into a Vitamix blender or food processor, and mix with other options.

Next, mix ½ cup oats into the blender or food processor. Oats will add more protein, fiber, and help thicken a smoothie.

For extra protein and fiber, add ⅓ cup chia seeds, ground flaxseed, sesame seeds, or hemp hearts.

- Chocolate flavor two tablespoons cocoa (or cacao, or carob) powder.

- Vanilla flavor, use ½ teaspoon of pure vanilla extract, the scrapings of ¼ of a vanilla bean, or ½ teaspoon vanilla powder.

- Coffee flavor, add one tablespoon instant espresso powder.

- Fruit flavors, add dried fruits of your liking to the mixture.

Grind the mixture until it becomes a smooth powder. Store the protein powder in an airtight container or jar and store in the fridge. For smoothies, use about two tablespoons of protein powder in a smoothie recipe.

Chapter 21: Foods to Eat for Increased Bone Healing

If you want to rebuild bones that represent the foundation and the fundamental structure of the human body, you need to give it the supplies it needs to build something that is going to last and speed up the healing process. Without proper diet and exercise, bone density deteriorates over time, leading to symptoms such as stooping, back pain, and fractures.

Restricting calories or not eating healthy during bone formation will slow the healing process. Your body will waste energy processing artificial foods, processed foods, unhealthy fats, oils, sugars, and gluten that it does not require to build your bone. The idea is to streamline the process and make your body work as little as possible on processing items it does not need in rebuilding your bones. The way you can do that is to give your body exactly what it needs and limit the intake of foods that slow the healing process.

Not only will you heal your bones, but your overall health will also increase substantially as your body thrives under the provided optimal conditions. With ideal nutrition and exercise, you stand to benefit from a speedy recovery.

BEST Anti-Inflammatory Foods.

- Dark chocolate has compounds called flavanols, which are packed with antioxidants that reduce inflammation.

- Cherries have antioxidants called anthocyanins and catechins, which fight inflammation.

- Grapes contain anthocyanins and resveratrol, which reduces inflammation. These antioxidants decrease inflammatory gene markers, including NF-kB

- Berries, including strawberries, blueberries, raspberries, and blackberries contain antioxidants called anthocyanins. These compounds are known to be anti-inflammatory.

- Fatty fish, such as salmon, sardines, herring, mackerel, and anchovies are high in long-chain omega-3 fatty acids EPA and DHA. EPA and DHA reduce inflammation after surgery or during the healing process.

- Turmeric has powerful anti-inflammatory nutrient curcumin. Turmeric is effective at reducing the inflammation related to arthritis, and other diseases.

- Extra virgin olive oil has a compound called oleocanthal, an antioxidant that is comparable to anti-inflammatory drugs like ibuprofen. Extra virgin olive oil has much higher anti-inflammatory benefits than refined olive oils.

- Avocados contain carotenoids and tocopherols, which reduce inflammation and lower levels of the inflammatory markers NF-kB and IL-6.

- Cruciferous vegetables, such as cauliflower, brussels sprouts, broccoli, and kale are high in antioxidants that are anti-inflammatory. Broccoli, for example, is high in sulforaphane, an antioxidant that lowers inflammation by reducing levels of cytokines and NF-kB, which causes inflammation.

- Green tea has a compound called epigallocatechin-3-gallate (EGCG). EGCG inhibits inflammation by reducing pro-inflammatory cytokine production and damage to the fatty acids in your cells. For an even more concentrated version, try matcha green tea powder, rich in catechins. This powerful antioxidant helps neutralize free radicals, harmful compounds that damage cells and cause chronic disease. The catechins in matcha are up to 137 times greater than in other types of green tea.

- Ginger has powerful anti-inflammatory and antioxidant properties.

- Rosemary is a rich source of antioxidants and anti-inflammatory compounds, which boost the immune system and improve blood circulation.

Best Foods for Strong Bones

- Vegetables, especially leafy greens, roots, and stalks provide iron, calcium, vitamin K, and C which works together with proteins to deposit collagen matrix (framework)

- Vegetables such as kale, collard greens, mustard greens, arugula, bok choy, parsley, pursalane, watercress, mesclun, broccoli, cabbage, carrots, zucchini, acorn, and butternut squash are high in calcium, magnesium, potassium, iron, and other minerals.

- Spinach and swiss chard are high in calcium, but are also high in oxalates which interfere with calcium absorption

- Seaweed, nuts, and seeds are foods rich in trace minerals. Having the proper balance of trace minerals can be more important than eating enough calcium.

- Plant-based proteins such as beans and soy, as well as animal-based proteins, for the collagen matrix.

- Proteins are what give bones their flexibility so they don't fracture. Plant-based protein sources leech less calcium from the body than animal-based proteins.

- Sardines have edible bones that provide calcium and other minerals.

- Whole grains are high in magnesium

- Eating 1 cup of whole grains per meal such as brown rice, millet, barley, buckwheat, oats, rye, amaranth, quinoa, and teff will provide the calories you'll need to repair bone, sparing the need to metabolize protein for energy

- Healthy fats for the fat-soluble vitamins needed such as vitamin K and D. Eating healthy fats boosts bone health

- Bone broth made by slow cooking bones with veggies, allows minerals to permeate into the vegetables.

Top 6 Ways to Drink Calcium

1. 1 cup fortified soymilk (160 mg), not fortified (19 mg)

2. 1 cup of fortified almond milk (160 mg), not fortified (0 mg)

3. 1 cup of cow's milk (300 mg)

4. 1 cup of rice milk (283 mg)

5. 1 cup of coconut milk (41 mg)

6. 1 cup of goat's milk (300 mg)

Top 5 Non-Dairy sources of calcium

1. Fish and shellfish

2. Soy products

3. Beans and legumes

4. Dark green leafy greens (including sea vegetables)

5. Nuts and seeds

Bone Broth

Bone broth is a soup made from cooking animal bones and connective tissues. It is good for the joints and digestive system and can be made from cow, pork, chicken, or fish bones. It contains vital nutrients and minerals.

The bones are simmered in water with vinegar to help release nutrients from the marrow as well as break down other tissues. The connective tissues contain collagen. Gelatin, which is formed from cooking collagen, provides the body with amino acids, which are the building blocks of proteins.

Some nutrients found in bone broth:

- calcium

- magnesium

- phosphorous

- iron

- vitamins A and K

- fatty acids

- selenium

- zinc

- manganese

Seven Benefits of Bone Broth:

1. Protects the joints

2. Source of gelatin which helps protect the joints.

3. Helps fight osteoarthritis

4. It improves joint symptoms, such as pain, stiffness, and decreased physical function in people with osteoarthritis.

5. It helps reduce inflammation and heal the gut.

6. Improves sleep

7. Supports weight loss

How to Make Bone Broth

Save the bones and cartilage from other meals or get them from your butcher.

1 gallon of water

1 ounce of vinegar

3–4 pounds of bones and tissues

- Boil the ingredients together in a large stockpot then simmer for 10–24 hours before letting it cool.

- Strain through a cheesecloth and store in smaller containers in the freezer.

- Heat these smaller containers as needed so the broth will last longer

- You can flavor with salt, vegetables, and spices to give the broth more flavor.

For joint pain and inflammation drink 2-4 cups of bone broth per day. If you just had surgery or if you're in an acute phase of an injury, drink 4 cups per day for 1-2 weeks to lower inflammation quickly.

Another option to liquid bone broth is bone broth powder, which typically is not as nutritionally rich, but much more convenient to use. Take 1-2 servings of the powder daily.

Gelatin

Gelatin is made by boiling animal bones, cartilage, and skin to extract the collagen. Collagen is a fibrous protein that connects muscles, bones, and skin in animals. Although gelatin is typically eaten as a dessert it is mostly made up of protein. Unlike collagen, the gelatin will dissolve in hot water, and is often used in soups, sauces, and desserts because of its texture.

Benefits of gelatin include:

- Gelatin contains several amino acids. Amino acids are used to make proteins, and are essential for building muscle, proper functioning of organs, and for providing energy. The most abundant amino acids in gelatin include glycine, proline, valine, lysine, alanine, and arginine. Valine is an essential amino acid that cannot be produced by the human body, which means it must come from the diet.

- Gelatin is used in medications, cosmetics as a gelling agent, gummy candies, marshmallows, and the coating of drug capsules.

- Collagen is what gives skin its healthy and youthful appearance. As people age, they naturally lose collagen which causes the skin to sag, wrinkle, and form crow's feet. Gelatin is a great source of collagen, and it may be a natural way to improve the skin's appearance.

- Gelatin provides protein, a macronutrient, which the body needs a large amount of

- Gelatin is a protein source that is fat-free.

- Gelatin is a digestive aid. It stimulates the production of gastric juices which facilitates proper digestion. Without adequate digestive enzymes, gastrointestinal problems, such as acid reflux, can develop. Gelatin also binds to water and helps food move through the digestive system efficiently.

- The collagen in gelatin decreases joint pain associated with inflammation. Gelatin reduces pain and improves joint function in people with osteoarthritis.

- Glycine, one of the most abundant amino acids in gelatin, improves blood sugar control in people with type 2 diabetes.

- Gelatin improves sleep quality due to the abundance of glycine.

- Lysine, which is found in gelatin, helps strengthen the bones. It helps the body absorb calcium, which helps keep bones strong and prevent bone loss. The body cannot make lysine; therefore, it must be obtained through the diet. Gelatin is a healthy way to increase your lysine intake.

- Due to its protein and low-calorie content, gelatin helps people feel full, which decreases the likelihood of overeating.

- The healthier the animal that is used to make gelatin, the higher the quality of the collagen.

- Homemade gelatin can be made by cooking bones of fish, poultry, pork, or beef for several hours. After the broth cools, you'll see a gel-substance on the surface, which is the collagen.

- Gelatin can be added to soups, stews, broths, sauces, mousse, and smoothies. Capsules or powders can be taken as a supplement by those who do not want to prepare the gelatin.

- Collagen peptides are identical to gelatin in their amino acid profiles, except that the chains of amino acids in collagen peptides have been cut into smaller pieces through hydrolysis. Collagen peptides also do not have the gelling functionality of gelatin and are soluble in cold water. In contrast, gelatin is used for its gelling properties, with many culinary uses and applications. As a result, collagen peptides are commonly used as a nutritional supplement. Because you can add it to your beverages or mix it into soups and sauces without changing their consistency.

Plant-based bone broth alternative.

Ingredients
12 cups of filtered water
1 tbsp coconut amino acids

1 extra-virgin olive oil or tbsp coconut oil
1 heaping tbsp of ginger, roughly chopped (with skins)
1 garlic bulb, crushed
1 red onion, quartered (with skins)
1 chili pepper, roughly chopped (with seeds)
1 tbsp peppercorns
3-4 cup mixed chopped vegetables and peelings, such as fresh mushrooms, carrot peelings, red cabbage, celery, and leeks
1 cup greens, such as spinach, chard, or kale
1/2 cup dried shiitake mushrooms
30 g dried wakame seaweed
2 tbsp ground turmeric (for a milder taste use less)
1/4 cup nutritional yeast flakes, for flavoring and vitamins
1 bunch of parsley, or other herbs of your choice

Instructions

Mix everything in a large pot, bring to a boil, and simmer with the lid on for about an hour.
Once everything has been cooked down, strain the liquid into a large bowl.

Serve immediately with some fresh herbs (cilantro, basil, etc.) for decoration or cool for later. It also freezes well.

Chapter 22: Supplements to Take for Increased Bone Healing

Recommended Daily Supplement for Bone Health

These are recommended daily amounts that can vary substantially depending on the factors that determine your bone mineral density (BMD). Your age, weight, sex, and lifestyle influence the number of nutrients needed to heal your bones quickly. However, it is important not to over supplement on any of the vital nutrients. It is suggested that you supplement within the recommended range and then eat the foods that are high in each of the nutrients. Your body will extract what it needs to complete the bone-building process.

Vitamins	
Folate (Folic Acid) (B9)	400 mcg
Vitamin B6 (Pyridoxine)	5-25 mg
Vitamin B12	1,000 mcg
Vitamin C	2,000 mg
Vitamin D	4,000 IU
Vitamin K	100-300 mcg
CoQ10	100-300 mg
Minerals	
Calcium	1,000-1,300 mg
Chromium	200 mcg
Boron	3 mg
Copper	2.5-10 mg

Magnesium	600 mg
Manganese	5-10 mg
Selenium	200 mcg
Silicon	1-2 mg
Strontium	0.5-3 mg
Zinc	50-100 mg
Phosphorus	700-1,200mg
Molybdenum	45 mcg
Fluoride	Do not supplement

Test your Microbiome

If you have a gut feeling something is slowing your healing, you could be right.

The gut microbiome can determine why some people heal much faster than others. Researchers found your gut bacteria, collectively known as your microbiome, can affect your ability to heal by influencing the absorption of nutrients and digestion of food. The bacteria studied were found to determine how well people can absorb nutrients in food and whether fiber and starches get broken down fast enough not to influence body healing.

Your gut microbiome is the types and numbers of microscopic organisms ("microbes") in your gastrointestinal (GI) tract. These include bacteria, fungi, viruses, parasites, and more. One method of determining your gut microbiome is testing stool samples. Your doctor can do this for you, or you can purchase an at-home stool testing kit (around $100). The test can reveal the types of microbes in your GI tract, as well as signs of inflammation that can cause health problems, food sensitivities, and digestive disorders.

These tests can help you figure out if you're eating the correct diet for your body's microbiome and, if not, what you should include to meet your dietary needs. In general, eating fiber-rich, plant-based, whole foods, not eating processed foods, and reducing animal protein intake are good for your microbiome.

Vitamins

Folate (Folic Acid) (B9)

Folic acid is a B vitamin, also known as folate (its related anion form), or as vitamin B9. Folate detoxifies a protein called homocysteine, an amino acid linked with bone inflammation and increased fracture risk. Homocysteine is released as you breakdown protein, therefore the more protein you include in your diet the more folate you'll need. As you age your body will produce more homocysteine which leads to osteoporosis. Folate will help prevent this, as well as prevent the formation of plaque in the arteries. Folate is not stored in the body, therefore, you must ingest some every day in your diet. Alcohol and birth control pills can prevent the absorption of folate.

Folate is also essential in preventing heart disease, strokes, chronic fatigue syndrome, infertility, depression, and birth defects such as neural tube defects and spina bifida. It is also essential in forming red blood cells, and genetic material such as RNA, and DNA.

Foods Rich in B9: beans, citrus fruits, whole grains, green leafy vegetables, beets, cauliflower, lettuce, asparagus.

Vitamin B6 (Pyridoxine)

B6 is used to produce the bone-building hormone progesterone and supports the protein structure of bones. Older people, people on high protein diets, and smokers are more likely to be deficient in this vitamin which causes bone fractures to heal slowly. B6 works with folate to metabolize homocysteine which protects the bones and

95

heart.

B6 helps with red blood cell formation, carpal tunnel syndrome, asthma, infertility, and osteoarthritis.

Foods Rich in B6: nuts (hazelnuts), eggs, pork, liver, brewer's yeast, whole grains (wheat, barley, buckwheat, rice), seafood (tuna, salmon, shrimp), chicken, beef, legumes (soybeans, chickpeas, black-eyed peas, pinto beans), sunflower seeds, lentils, tomato, avocado, vegetables (cauliflower, watercress, kale, kohlrabi, brussels sprouts, onions, okra, broccoli, squash, spinach, garden cress, carrots, radishes).

Vitamin B12 (Cobalamin)

B12 works with folate and B6 to protect against the effects of homocysteine. B6 is essential for red blood cell formation, protecting nerve fibers, cell division, and DNA formation. B12 levels decrease with age, so supplementation needs to increase to compensate.

Foods Rich in B12: Yeast, tempeh, miso, soy sauce, milk, eggs, dairy, fish (herring, flounder, sardines, mackerel), liver, and beef.

Vitamin C (Ascorbate, Ascorbic Acid and L-Ascorbic Acid)

Vitamin C is necessary for the formation of cartilage, collagen, boosts the immune system, heals wounds, cuts, bruises, and assists with calcium absorption. Vitamin C is an antioxidant that helps with the absorption of iron, metabolizing proteins, and protects cells from damage.

Foods Rich in Vitamin C: Vegetables (brussels sprouts, sweet potatoes, snow peas, potatoes, broccoli, cauliflower, peas, kale), fruits (guava, cantaloupe, papaya, citrus fruits, strawberries, tomatoes)

Vitamin D (D3 (Cholecalciferol) and D2 (Ergocalciferol)

Vitamin D is the second most important nutrient for bone healing after calcium. Vitamin D3 is used for the synthesis of calcium. Without Vitamin D you would not absorb and properly balance calcium and phosphorus. Vitamin D also lowers excessive levels of parathyroid hormone, which protects against bone loss. Most of the vitamin D your body makes is produced by exposure to sunlight. Your body uses the sun's ultraviolet (UV) rays to convert cholesterol in your skin to vitamin D. If you live somewhere where the days are shorter, spend most of your time indoors, or have a darker skin color, you will have to monitor how much vitamin D you're getting to make sure you're getting enough. Dark skin color is nature's sunblock, the darker your skin color the more melanin in your skin. This additional pigmentation will give you extra protection from the sun, but it also limits the amount of vitamin D your body can produce because it limits UV light absorption, whereas a person with lighter skin color may be able to get enough vitamin D with just 20 minutes of sunlight a day. A person with a darker complexion will need more time in the sun, depending on how dark their skin is. This would be difficult to quantify without taking blood tests to measure how much vitamin D your body makes after sun exposure. Therefore, it is recommended that you take vitamin D supplements and get sunlight to help speed the healing process. If you're bed-bound go out into the sunlight in a wheelchair and expose your limbs to the sunlight. You can keep your face covered if you're concerned about wrinkles, however, your limbs must be exposed to direct sunlight to get the benefits. Do not wear sunblock on your limbs to maximize the production of vitamin D

Calciferol (ergocalciferol) also known as vitamin D2, is used to treat hypoparathyroidism, rickets, and low levels of phosphate in the blood.

Insufficient amounts of vitamin D can lead to soft bones, osteomalacia, rickets, or osteoporosis. Vitamin D also needs fats to be absorbed, therefore low-fat diets can also cause bone problems.

Vitamin D is also good for the prevention of colon and breast cancer and lowering blood pressure. Anticonvulsant medications can deplete vitamin D levels.

Foods Rich in Vitamin D: Fortified dairy, bread, and cereals. Fish (sardines, tuna, mackerel, salmon, and herring), fish liver oils, eel, avocado, organ meats, and egg yolks.

Vitamin K (Phylloquinone)

Vitamin K activates osteocalcin, which is a protein crucial in the bone matrix. Osteocalcin is second to collagen in importance, without it your bones would be like chalk. Vitamin K attracts calcium and holds it in place.

Vitamin K is normally made in the intestines and is also important in clotting blood, maintaining the cell membrane, and fat synthesis. Antibiotic treatments can destroy the bacteria which leads to damage to the bones.

Foods Rich in Vitamin K: Green leafy vegetables (kale, spinach, turnip greens, collards, Swiss chard, mustard greens, parsley, romaine, and green leaf lettuce),

vegetables (brussels sprouts, broccoli, cauliflower, and cabbage), fish, liver, meat, and eggs.

CoQ10 (Ubiquinone)

Coenzyme Q10 (CoQ10) is an antioxidant that your body produces naturally. Your body's cells use CoQ10 for growth and maintenance. It protects cells from damage and plays an important part in metabolism and therefore aids in the body's healing after surgery and in healing broken bones.

Foods Rich in CoQ10: CoQ10 is found naturally in food, but in quantities lower than what can be obtained through supplements. Good food sources of CoQ10 include: tuna, salmon, mackerel, sardines, vegetable oils, and meats

Minerals

Calcium (Ca)

Calcium carbonate is the most common form of calcium found in over-the-counter (OTC) antacid products. Calcium citrate is the second most common form of calcium found. Other types of calcium include; gluconate, lactate, and phosphate. When taken with food, they have all shown to be equally effective and absorbed.

Calcium helps your muscles, nerves, and cells work normally. Calcium is the main ingredient in bones, and bones are the main storage area for calcium. Your body's calcium requirements must be met through your diet as your body is unable to make calcium. Without sufficient amounts of calcium in your diet, your bones can become weak and will not grow properly.

Only 15% to 20% of the calcium you eat will be absorbed in your gut. Vitamin D helps the gut absorb more calcium, therefore, low vitamin D levels cause an increased risk for fractures.

Hormonal signals take some calcium out of the bones every day to keep blood calcium levels normal, release hormones, maintain blood Ph, move blood through the body, move muscles, allow nerves to carry messages between the brain and all parts of the body, and enzymes that affect almost every function in the human body.

People that consume large amounts of sodium in their diets through processed, canned, or any other type of high sodium food, are at risk for losing calcium which is extracted from the body as the kidneys excrete sodium.

Foods Rich in Calcium: Seeds, fish (sardines, salmon), beans and lentils, almonds, rhubarb, oranges, seaweed, parsley, leafy greens, and dairy products. If you're going to eat dairy products use organic, raw, full-fat whole milk without synthetic vitamin D, unpasteurized cheese, and yogurt made from whole milk from organic grass-fed cows. Fermented milk products that have lost their lactose are the easiest to assimilate. While milk is fortified with vitamin D, most other dairy products are not. Yogurt is very high in calcium, while cottage cheese is very low.

Boron (B)

Boron is essential to endocrine function which helps activate vitamin D, and maintain the balance of calcium and magnesium. Without enough boron, your bones can become brittle, and essential chemical reactions throughout your body will not take place.

Foods Rich in Boron; seeds (almonds, poppy, cumin seeds, hazelnuts, and peanuts), nuts (pistachios), fruit (apples, oranges, prunes, pears, strawberries, cherries, apricots, grapes, figs, currants, raisins, peaches), honey, legumes (beans, soybeans, and peas), vegetables (onions, parsley, cabbage, asparagus, broccoli, tomatoes, beets, leafy vegetables), and herbs including dill, stinging nettle, and dandelion.

Copper (Cu)

Copper is responsible for the cross-linking of collagen and elastin in the organic bone matrix which gives bone strength. Therefore, it slows bone breakdown and assists in repairs. Deficiency inhibits bone growth, causes skeletal abnormalities, fragility, and promotes pathological changes characteristic of osteoporosis. Copper is also essential in the creation of red blood cells and heart muscle function.

Food Rich in Copper; green leafy vegetables, legumes (especially peas), poultry, eggs, shellfish, whole grains, nuts, and organ meats especially liver.

Copper bracelets will supplement copper transdermally through your skin. As your body reaches adequate copper levels it will stop absorbing the copper and your skin will start to turn green. Although the green color is unsightly it is harmless.

Magnesium (Mg)

The third most crucial nutrient for bone mineral density (BMD). Over 75% of people are deficient in magnesium. As you age your body has difficulty absorbing magnesium. Magnesium gives bones their structural strength. Magnesium also plays a role in controlling parathyroid hormone, estrogen, calcitonin levels in the body, normal body weight, lowering high blood pressure, and lowering high cholesterol. Magnesium controls respiratory disorders such as bronchitis, asthma, wheezing. counters PMS symptoms, mental illness, depression, hallucinations, agitation, headaches, bursitis, angina, irregular heartbeat, irritable bowel syndrome, arteriosclerosis, heart attacks, gum disease, tendonitis, and reduces the likelihood of recurrent kidney stones. Taking calcium and magnesium supplements before bedtime can help prevent nighttime leg cramps. Lack of magnesium can cause nausea and muscle weakness. Alcohol consumption causes decreased absorption of magnesium, which causes depletion of bone calcium.

The best type of magnesium supplement to take is magnesium citrate which has a high bioavailability and is easily absorbed. Taking high levels of calcium, but low levels of magnesium can cause bone loss. Keep calcium to magnesium supplements at a 2 to 1 ratio. Taking too much magnesium can cause diarrhea. Don't take magnesium supplements if you're on a renal diet.

Foods Rich in Magnesium: Green leafy vegetables (spinach, lettuce, chard), green vegetables (celery, green beans), milk, whole grains (oats, wheat germ), fish and seafood, brown rice, seeds (poppy, pumpkin, and sunflower), nuts (brazil, almonds, and cashews), fruits (bananas, avocados), legumes (soybeans, peas, red beans, black beans, and black eye peas), dark chocolate, quinoa, molasses, and herbs such as; dandelion, licorice root, coriander, stinging nettle, and purslane.

Manganese (Mn)

Manganese is essential in the formation of parts of the bone, cartilage, and the matrix structure to which calcium attaches to. It is also essential for activating the enzymes that enable chemical reactions throughout the body. Deficiency in manganese will affect sex hormone production which affects bone formation and exacerbates bone loss.

Foods Rich in Manganese: Nuts (almonds and pecans), legumes (lima and pinto beans), whole grains (oatmeal, bran cereals, whole wheat, brown rice), leafy green vegetables (spinach), fruits (pineapple and acai), tea, dark chocolate.

Selenium (Se)

Selenium is critical to various enzymatic reactions throughout the body and is one of the building blocks of the bone matrix. Selenium is an antioxidant that works with vitamin E to prevent breast cancer. It is also an antiviral agent, slows the progression of cataracts, and prevents damage to organs and cells. A deficiency in selenium has been linked to heart failure and heart abnormalities.

Foods Rich in Selenium: Brazil nuts, sunflower seeds, fish (tuna, salmon, sardines, oysters, mussels), pork, beef, turkey, chicken, garlic, cucumbers, onions, mushrooms, whole grains (wheat and oat bran)

Silicon (Si)

Silicon supports calcification and is important for the formation of connective tissue, cartilage, and tendons. With age and decreased hormone production, silicon levels decrease and arthritis becomes more prevalent.

Silicon supplementation is good for balding, kidney stones, urinary tract health, tendonitis, fractures, arthritis, and bursitis. Homeopathic silica supplements improve bone nutrition and growth.

Foods Rich in Silicon: Nuts (cashews, walnuts, brazil nuts, pistachios), brown rice, cucumbers, barley, turnips, string beans, and the herbs horsetail, stinging nettle, and chickweed.

Strontium (Sr)

Necessary for bone remodeling and helps attract calcium to bones. Strontium helps in the treatment of arthritis and bone pain.

Foods Rich in Strontium: Plants are better sources of strontium than meats, but it depends on the quality of the soil where the food was grown. Strontium is found in whole grains, spices, legumes, root and leafy vegetables, and seafood.

Zinc (Zn)

Zinc is vital in the formation of osteoblasts, osteoclasts, bone proteins, assists in repairs, and vitamin D function. Zinc is vital to healthy hair, shortening PMS cycles, shortening colds, prostate health, stress, and wound healing.

Foods Rich in Zinc: egg yolks, seeds (pumpkin, sesame, sunflower), legumes, beef, pork, lamb, poultry, crab, fish, dairy, oysters

Phosphorus (P)

Phosphorus works with calcium to help build bones, nucleic acids, and cell membranes. It's also involved in the body's energy production. If calcium levels are too high your body absorbs less phosphorus. You also need vitamin D to absorb phosphorus properly. Phosphorus is found in almost all foods so it's difficult to not get enough of it in your diet. Excess phosphorus, however, can prevent calcium absorption. Drinking soft drinks, eating large amounts of meat, and grains can cause an oversupply of phosphorus.

Foods Rich in Phosphorus: tuna, pork chops, tofu, dairy, chicken, scallops, lentils, squash, pumpkin seeds, beef, beer, quinoa.

Molybdenum (Mo)

Molybdenum prevents the build-up of deadly sulfites and toxins and is critical to various enzymatic reactions throughout the body.

Foods Rich in Molybdenum: Navy beans, almonds, soy, dairy,

Fluoride (F)

Fluoride combines with calcium in the bone and prevents bone loss. Being deficient in naturally occurring fluoride will cause osteoporosis. Most people will get enough fluoride from municipal water and food. However, most people overdose with fluoride, so do not supplement it. In fact, for your overall health, it is better to avoid any products (toothpaste, mouthwash, and teeth whiteners) with fluoride. Over supplementing fluoride can cause fluorosis, neurological, skeletal, and thyroid problems.

Foods Rich in Fluoride: tea, tap water, wine, raisins, shrimp, and blue crab.

Chapter 23: Herbal Remedies for Increased Bone Healing

12 Herbs to Increase Bone Health

1. Alfalfa; can be used as a treatment for asthma, arthritis, diabetes, blood sugar control, excessive production of urine (diuresis), relieving symptoms of menopause high cholesterol, indigestion, and excessive bruising or bleeding. Alfalfa is high in antioxidants, vitamins C and K, copper, folate and magnesium.

2. Anise; helps improve digestion, constipation, gas, bloating, alleviate cramps, reduce nausea, and for treating cough and flu. Anise is rich in iron and manganese

3. Bayberry Bark; used to treat head colds, painful and swollen intestines (colitis), vomiting, diarrhea, nausea, and to stimulate the circulatory system.

4. Black Currant Seed; Black currant seed oil contains gamma-linolenic acid (GLA), an omega-6 fatty acid that helps ease inflammation in the body. Black currant seed also helps treat joint pain, stiffness, soreness, and damage.

5. Oil Blessed Thistle; used for loss of appetite, indigestion, colds, cough, fever, bacterial infections, diarrhea, a diuretic to increase urine output, and for promoting the flow of breast milk in new mothers.

6. Blue Cohosh; used to treat symptoms of menopause, premenstrual syndrome (PMS), painful menstruation, weakened bones (osteoporosis), acne, and starting labor in pregnant women.

7. Burdock Root; contains multiple types of powerful antioxidants, including quercetin, luteolin, and phenolic acids, removes toxins from the blood, inhibits some types of cancer, maybe an aphrodisiac, and treats skin disorders.

8. Cramp (viburnum) Bark; contains ellagic acid, which has antioxidants, and is used to treat arthritis, chronic pain, high blood pressure, inflammation, low back pain, menopausal symptoms, menstrual cramps, and restless legs syndrome.

9. Damian; used to treat headache, bedwetting, depression, nervous stomach, constipation, headaches, weight loss, for prevention and treatment of sexual problems, boosting and maintaining mental and physical stamina, and as an aphrodisiac.

10. Motherwort; used for heart conditions, anxiety, absence of menstrual periods, intestinal gas, and hyperthyroidism.

11. Pennyroyal; used for colds, pneumonia, other breathing problems, stomach pains, gas, intestinal disorders, liver, and gallbladder problems. Pennyroyal is also used to kill germs, repel insects, treat skin diseases, topically for gout, venomous bites, and for mouth sores.

12. Slippery Elm; used for coughs, sore throat, colic, diarrhea, constipation, hemorrhoids, irritable bowel syndrome (IBS), bladder and urinary tract infections, syphilis, herpes, and for expelling tapeworms. Slippery elm coats and soothes the mouth, throat, stomach, and intestines.

Herbs Rich in Calcium

1. Chaya: Chaya (Cnidoscolus chayamansa) is a shrub native to Mexico's Yucatan peninsula. It is also known as tree spinach. Chaya has more protein, calcium, iron, vitamin C, and carotenes than spinach. The leaves are used to treat obesity, kidney stones, hemorrhoids, acne, and eye problems. It is also used to stimulate circulation, improve digestion, strengthen fingernails, and as a laxative and diuretic. Chaya leaves contain hydrocyanic glycosides, which are toxic compounds, but are easily destroyed by cooking. Chaya is cooked for 20 minutes and served with butter or oil. Don't cook chaya in an aluminum pot, or it can cause a toxic reaction that can result in diarrhea.

2. Comfrey: Comfrey is a shrub that grows in parts of Europe, Asia, and North America. It was initially called "knit bone" and people used it to treat muscle sprains, bruises, burns, joint inflammation, back pain, osteoarthritis, gout, and to treat diarrhea and other stomach ailments.

The roots or leaves of the comfrey plant contain chemical substances called allantoin and rosmarinic acid. Allantoin speeds up wound healing by stimulating the growth of new skin cells, while rosmarinic acid helps relieve pain and has anti-inflammatory compounds. Comfrey is safe for most people when applied to unbroken skin in small amounts for less than ten days. It contains chemicals called pyrrolizidine alkaloids that can cause liver damage, lung damage, cancer, and even death when you consume them. Avoid taking comfrey by mouth or using it on open wounds.

3. Dandelion: Dandelion (Taraxacum officinale) is the same weed that grows on your lawn. It is used for treating cancer, anti-aging, boosting your immune system, reducing blood sugar, lowering blood pressure, reducing cholesterol, rebuilding broken bones, anti-inflammatory, acne, weight loss, liver disease, and digestive disorders. Dandelions greens can be eaten cooked or raw and is an excellent source of vitamins A, B, C, E, K, iron, calcium, magnesium, potassium, and fiber.

Dandelion can cause allergic reactions, particularly in people with allergies to related plants like ragweed. Contact dermatitis can also occur in people with sensitive skin.

Dandelion may interact unfavorably with some medications, especially certain diuretics and antibiotics.

4. Horsetail: The chemicals in horsetail have antioxidant and anti-inflammatory effects. Horsetail can reduce edema, kidney and bladder stones, urinary tract infections, the inability to control urination (incontinence), and general disturbances of the kidney and bladder. Also used for balding, tuberculosis, jaundice, hepatitis, brittle fingernails, joint diseases, gout, osteoarthritis, weak bones (osteoporosis), high cholesterol levels, frostbite, weight loss, heavy menstrual periods, and uncontrolled bleeding (hemorrhage) of the nose, lung, or stomach. Horsetail can be applied directly to the skin to treat wounds and burns.

5. Mugwort: Mugwort is a plant that grows in Asia, North America, and Northern Europe. It is used for treating menstrual problems, boosting energy, stomach and intestinal conditions including colic, diarrhea, constipation, cramps, weak digestion, worm infestations, persistent vomiting, and for stimulating gastric juice and bile secretion. It is also used as a liver tonic to promote circulation, as a sedative in the treatment of hysteria, epilepsy, and convulsions in children. Mugwort root treats mental problems, depression, hypochondria, irritability, restlessness, insomnia, and anxiety. Mugwort lotion can also be applied directly to the skin to relieve itchiness caused by burn scars.

6. Oatstraw: Oat straw extract comes from its stems and leaves, which are harvested earlier while the grass is still green. It's high in iron, manganese, and zinc. Some of the benefits include improved brain function, reduced inflammation, improved blood flow, insomnia, reduced anxiety, depression, stress, and physical and sexual performance.

7. Pigweed: Pigweed is high in vitamins A, C, manganese, calcium, and is high in magnesium, phosphorus, potassium, and zinc. It is used to treat profuse menstruation, intestinal bleeding, diarrhea, and hoarseness.

8. Plantain Leaves: The plantain plant, also known as Plantago lanceolata, has a worldwide distribution. It has bioactive compounds such as catalpol, aucubin, and acteoside. These compounds are anti-inflammatory, antioxidant, antineoplastic, and hepatoprotective. Plantain leaves are also used to treat cough, wounds, dermatitis, insect bites and stings, and eczema. It works as a pain reliever, antifungal, and anti-ulcerative.

Plantain leaves are high in vitamins A, C, K, calcium, iron, manganese, and potassium.

9. Purslane: Purslane is best known as a weed that grows in many parts of the world. However, it is also an edible and nutritious vegetable. Purslane is full of nutrients, including omega-3 fatty acids, glutathione, melatonin, and betalain. Purslane is high in vitamin A, C, E, magnesium, manganese, potassium, iron, calcium, vitamins B1, B2, B3, folate, copper, and phosphorus. It's one of the most nutritious plants you can eat. Purslane helps lower cholesterol, and is used in anti-aging, reducing abnormal uterine bleeding, asthma, type 2 diabetes, regulating blood pressure, lowering the risk of stroke and heart disease, and rebuilding bones. Purslane contains oxalates that are an antinutrient and cause kidney stones, so eat in small doses. Adding it to yogurt also reduces the number of oxalates.

10. Raspberry Leaves: Red raspberry is a plant native to Europe and parts of Asia, and is known for its sweet, nutritious berries. It is high in polyphenols like tannins and flavonoids, ellagic acids, vitamins B and C, potassium, magnesium, calcium, zinc, phosphorus and iron.

The leaves are used to induce labor, helps relieve premenstrual symptoms (PMS), such as cramping, vomiting, nausea, and diarrhea. It also contains fragarine, a plant compound that helps tone and tighten muscles in the pelvic area, which reduces the menstrual cramping caused by muscle spasms, and helps make delivery easier.

11. Red Clover: Red clover (Trifolium pratense) is typically used to treat asthma, whooping cough, bronchitis, eczema, psoriasis, heart disease, arthritis, cancer, cholesterol, osteoporosis, and menopause.

Red clover has calcium, chromium, magnesium, isoflavones, niacin, phosphorus, potassium, thiamine, and vitamin C.

12. Sage: Sage (salvia officinalis) is one of the most diverse herbs available and is used to treat digestive problems, loss of appetite, flatulence, gastritis, diarrhea, bloating, heartburn, improve memory, boost brain function, depression, diabetes, and lowers cholesterol. Sage has also been used to treat Alzheimer's disease, prevent lung cancer, asthma, reduce pain after surgery, and cerebral ischemia. Sage is used for painful menstrual periods, to correct excessive milk flow during nursing, to reduce hot flashes during menopause, cold sores, gingivitis, sore mouth, throat, or tongue, swollen, painful nasal passages, and swollen tonsils. It is also applied to the skin after sun exposure to prevent sunburn.

Sage is rich in vitamin A, B vitamins, K, magnesium, calcium, and phosphorus.

13. Stinging Nettle: Stinging nettle (urtica dioica) is used to treat arthritis, back pain, cancer, anti-aging, reduce inflammation, arthritis, prostatitis, hay fever, lower blood pressure, lower blood sugar, reduce bleeding after surgery, protect the liver, heal wounds and burns, and is used as a natural diuretic.

Stinging nettle is rich in vitamins A, C, K, B vitamins, calcium, iron, magnesium, phosphorus, potassium, sodium, linoleic acid, linolenic acid, palmitic acid, stearic acid, oleic acid, amino acids, and polyphenols.

14. Yellow Dock: Yellow dock is native to Europe and Asia. It is used to treat poor digestion, scurvy, intestinal infections, arthritis, jaundice, fungal infections, skin conditions, mild constipation, and as a liver detox.

Yellow Dock is rich in vitamins A, C, calcium, phosphorus, magnesium, potassium, silicon, iron, sulfur, copper, iodine, manganese, and zinc.

Herb Sources of Phytoestrogens:

Phytoestrogens are plant-based compounds that mimic estrogen in the body. Phytoestrogens play a role in preventing bone loss caused by estrogen deficiency by helping maintain calcium and vitamin D in your bones.

Herbs that are a good source of phytoestrogens include; Black Cohosh, Chaste tree (vitex), Dong Quai, Elder, False

Unicorn Root, Fennel, Fenugreek, Ginseng, Lady's Slipper, Licorice, Life root, Passionflower, Sarsaparilla, Sassafras, Unicorn Root, and Wild Yam Root Bark.

Chapter 24: Foods to Avoid for Increased Bone Healing

Factors That Deplete Calcium from Your Bones

- Too much or too little protein, or eating low quality protein

- An acid-alkaline imbalance will drain your bones of calcium. The body needs to have a slightly alkaline pH of 7.45 for ideal health.

- Eating acid forming foods such as sugar and high fructose corn syrup can deplete calcium from bones

- Eating sugary foods can cause an interference in calcium and magnesium absorption causing osteoporosis. Eating foods high in sugar can also lead to increased insulin levels, diabetes mellitus, elevated blood pressure, elevated cholesterol levels, cardiovascular disease, gallstones, obesity, mood swings, depression, increased stomach acid, weakened immune system, migraines, and depletion of copper, vitamin B, C.

- Low fat and fat free products are high in sugar and contain artificial ingredients

- Overconsumption of soy products has negative effects on estrogen levels which affects calcium absorption

- Caffeine causes damage to bone mineral density and increases risk of fractures. Caffeine consumption increases the excretion of calcium and magnesium through the urine resulting in bone loss. The following foods contain caffeine: coffee, tea, soda, energy drinks, and chocolate.

- Smoking causes decreased bone density due to decreased blood oxygen levels.

- Losing too much weight and being too thin will cause decreased bone mineral density.

- Eating refined carbohydrates such as white bread and pasta daily.

- Eating uncooked nightshade vegetables, such as tomatoes, goji berries, peppers, white potatoes, chili peppers, bell peppers, tomatillos, and eggplant. These foods slow the healing process, and can cause bone inflammation, which can lead to osteoporosis if eaten over a prolonged period of time.

- Taking lots of medication.

- Not going out in the sun.

- Not exercising or doing little if any exercise.

- Eating fresh foods will ensure higher levels of calcium.

- Try to cook food yourself from their raw forms, instead of using cans, boxes, frozen, or packaged foods which tend to have lower levels of calcium.

- Oxalates, found in vegetables such as Swiss chard, beet greens, and spinach, prevent calcium from being absorbed in the digestive tract. Cooking these vegetables destroys the oxalic acid and allows absorption of calcium, however, eating large quantities may cause kidney stones.

- Phytates also combine with calcium to produce a substance that can not be absorbed by the intestines. Foods that are high in phytates include beans, grains, nuts, and seeds. Phytates only affect the absorption of calcium if eaten in large quantities.

- Difficulty in absorbing fats may indicate difficulty in absorbing vitamin D which in turn leads to diminished calcium absorption.

- Exceeding 1000 milligrams of caffeine will lead to

difficulty in retaining calcium.

- Alcohol affects the body's ability to absorb vitamin D.

Warning Signs of Insufficient Calcium Intake;

- A white coating on the tongue, sticky sour taste in the mouth, and bad breath is a sign you may be eating too many acid-forming foods. These foods leach calcium from your bones to neutralize the acid.

- Problems with teeth and gums can mean problems with the mineral density of bones.

- Joint and back pain can also be a sign of decreased calcium absorption.

- Too much stress causes damage to the adrenal glands which causes an increase in cortical steroid levels which then increases the risk of osteoporosis.

- Other symptoms of inadequate calcium; loss of height, nocturnal leg cramps, transparent skin, rheumatoid arthritis, restless behavior (foot jiggling, and hair twisting), insomnia.

Guidelines When Eating Out;

1. Eat at least 1-2 salads a day. Use olive oil and lemon juice as a dressing. No fat-free dressings as they contain too many chemicals.

2. Eat proteins such as ocean fish, organic free-range chicken or beef. If you're vegetarian eat lots of bean dishes.

3. Avoid soups that are tomato, cream, or flour-based. Eat chicken, beef, barley, bean, and vegetable minestrone soups.

4. Eat 2-3 cooked vegetables with every meal such as cooked greens, squash, zucchini, broccoli, green beans, bok choy, and turnips.

5. Avoid vegetables in the nightshade family such as tomatoes, eggplant, bell pepper, and white potatoes.

6. Limit eating tomato-based sauces to only once a week.

7. Avoid caffeine, diet drinks, and soft drinks.

8. Avoid commercial desserts made with refined sugar and flour.

Best Food Options by Different Restaurant Types;

1. Coffee shops; Drink naturally caffeine-free drinks like peppermint and mint tea, water, or sparkling water. Avoid sweets. Eat salads, soups, and protein dishes.

2. Chinese restaurants; Request that sugar and msg not be added to your food. Request brown rice instead of white rice. Get stir-fried vegetables with different meats or tofu.

3. Italian restaurants; avoid pasta. Eat meat dishes and salads.

4. Upscale restaurants; Eat veggies and proteins; avoid deserts.

5. Mexican restaurants; Avoid chiles, tomato salsas, corn tortillas made from GMO corn, flour tortillas, chips, and cheese. Eat meat dishes, guacamole,

6. Japanese restaurants; Avoid tuna due to mercury, and teriyaki due to sugar. Eat dishes with seaweeds

7. Greek restaurants; Lamb, salads, olive oil

8. Indian restaurants; Eat vegetables and protein dishes

9. Fast food restaurants; Avoid due to msg, & trans fats.

Chapter 25: My Routine on How to Prepare for a Fast Recovery from a Bone Injury

The first thing to do is make a game plan based on the type of injury, expected recovery time, and your personal goals. When people get hurt, I often see them become passive and just accept that they're going to be out of commission for a prolonged period of time.

An injury is rarely expected, that's why they're called accidents and when it happens, you'll have a lot of work to do to prepare and be successful for the outcomes that await you. Focus on five areas; physical, social, spiritual, mental, and emotional. Don't worry about your past lifestyle. You can't change that, focus instead on the future and making changes to accelerate your healing.

Start by learning everything you can about your injury and studying how to treat it.

You'll have limited time when you see your doctors and therapists, and at the end of the treatment they'll ask, "Do you have any questions?" Most likely, you won't know what to ask and you won't understand everything said because you may not have a medical background. Keep in mind that your medical team is tasked with treating you, and it's your job to make sure you understand the process, and implement it. By understanding your injury, you'll know what precautions to take to avoid further injury, have knowledge of alternative or new treatments that may be available, what to expect, and what actions you can take on your own to treat and move your healing along quickly.

How to Use this Book

To write this book, I had to become this book. I tried multiple strategies and read thousands of research pages to develop this bone healing plan. According to seven of the best Los Angeles surgeons, my only survival option was amputation of my left leg. With over twenty years of experience working with people who have suffered some of the worst accidents, I knew this was not the life I wanted. I had to quickly discover and utilize the best treatment options for healing, or I would go bankrupt and live the rest of my life as an amputee. I wrote this book to help anyone who might be in the same situation I faced and who needed to heal as quickly as possible to get back to living their life. You create a healthier version of yourself by adapting your habits and lifestyle. Bad habits can be self-reinforcing; before you know it, everything you do helps you maintain your predicted diagnosis of permanent disability. For example, you wake up in the morning, and because you feel pain and can't walk, move your arm, or use whichever bone is broken, you decide to lie in bed because you can't use the broken bones. Well, you have many more bones in your body that need to be put to work, or your health begins to spiral downward. Everyone who feels sorry for you has already made you believe you have the right to mope, be sad, and do nothing. So this belief makes you feel entitled to lay in bed watching Netflix all day, so you no longer manage your diet or exercise. As you become weaker, you feel more sorry for yourself, which causes stress, and the stress causes more self-pity, weight gain, and disability. So the disability cycle continues and often worsens as we mature and develop more habits that support the disabled version of ourselves.

Start by thinking about the person you want to become and the ideal condition you want to be in. Put a picture of yourself of when you were in your best shape or a picture of someone who looks how you want to look and post it close to your bed, so you look at it every time you wake up and go to bed to remind yourself of your goal.

Lee Robins completed a research study on heroin-addicted soldiers after the Vietnam War. Robins' studies found that over 99% of people that returned from Vietnam recovered because they were in a new environment. Whereas when people come out of rehab and go back home, over 90% fail because they're returning to the same domain and stimulus that caused the addiction in the first place. So for anyone in a funk, it's crucial that you completely

117

change the setting and for them to change their routines.

Wearing a cast will not immediately heal your broken bones. But if the goal is to become whole again and you identify as an entire person (no broken bones), you will do the necessary work to become healed. So if you cook something healthy, So if you cook something healthy, that does not make you healthy. However, believing that you are healthy will lead to choosing and eating healthier foods.

Everyone wants to become a millionaire, but not everyone becomes a millionaire. So everyone has the same goal, but they don't have the same methodology, so you have to develop the method to reach the same goal as the actual millionaires.

The second step will consist of getting a notebook and writing down your daily routine with the foods you eat and the activities you engage in throughout your typical day. Research shows that writing things down will keep you motivated, help you learn, and encourages daily progress. Analyzing your habits is essential because they help you become the person you want to be (healthy), not because of outcomes such as a better body. Even though that may be the outcome of your behavior changes, as you read this book, start with the suggestions that are most appealing or easiest for you to start using. Reference your daily routine and write where you will add in, subtract, or swap behaviors in your daily routine. As you make changes to your daily routine, rewrite the new routine on the next page and keep everything in your notebook so you can reference back to your changes in the future.

For example, you are swapping coconut oil for vegetable oils. So you change your environment by removing the vegetable oils in your home and replacing them with coconut oil. That will be the only option available when you cook, and you remove the temptation of using vegetable oils. Think about being in the office, and someone brings a box of donuts in the morning. You say no because you don't want the extra calories, but as the day goes on and you see the donuts throughout the day, your willpower starts to weaken, and by the end of the day, you rationalize eating a donut because you don't want them to go to waste.

The goal is to give herself some new structure so you can follow a general direction. But still, allow for flexibility, creativity, and spontaneity to enjoy your day. No daily routine is perfect, and as you adjust, if you feel like you cannot complete a portion of your routine, you should swap it out for something else. Spend time designing and changing your routine or systems to lead to better outcomes and meet your goals instead of just focusing on your goals.

As you adjust your routine, eliminate your negative self-talk. Otherwise, you'll only be reinforcing the behavior you are trying to change. Making 1% changes a month will lead to a 37% improvement a year. Missing one day or participating in a bad habit one time will not affect you. The gradual accumulation of those good or bad habits makes a difference.

However, be as consistent as possible so that it becomes predictable and your body has a biological clock to initiate it. Such as, I wake up in the morning and drink three glasses of water instead of saying I'm going to drink more water, and I have no idea about the time and place you're going to do it. That's predictability, so it becomes automatic. Also, be specific such as when I open my eyes, I drink the water. Mention each trigger for each habit sequentially.

Psychoacoustic Medicine

In the 1980s, the CIA developed a top-secret training system called the Gateway Experience that uses sounds (binaural beats) to manipulate brain waves to enhance strength, focus, manifest goals, convert energy to heal one's body, and even travel across space and time to access new information. This technique has been expanded into Psychoacoustic Medicine, where music and sound facilitate your nervous system into changing your psychological and physiological state. Binaural beats are created by the brain when you simultaneously listen to different tones in each ear with headphones. The two tones align with your brain waves to produce a beat with a different frequency. This is the hertz (Hz) difference between the two tones' frequencies. Your brain deciphers the two tones as a different beat and will match the frequency set by the frequency of the sound, the frequency-following effect. For example, if you listen to a 444 Hz tone with your right ear and a 440 Hz tone with your left ear, you would hear a 4 Hz tone. Specific binaural beat frequencies train your mind to increase or decrease brain functions that control thinking, healing, weight loss, and feeling.

Five brain waves create binaural beats and lead to different mental states.

A. Gamma: 30-100 Hz: Increased cognitive enhancement, Attention to detail and memory recall, Creativity

B. Beta: 14-30 Hz: Keeping your attention focused, Analytical thinking and solving problems, Stimulating energy and action, High-level cognition

C. Alpha: 8-14 Hz: Relax and focus, Reduce Stress, Maintain positive thinking, Increase your learning capabilities

D. Theta: 4-8 Hz: Meditation, Deep relaxation, Creativity

E. Delta: 1-4 Hz: Deep sleep, Healing and pain relief, Meditation, Anti-aging: cortisol reduction/DHEA increase, Access to the unconscious mind

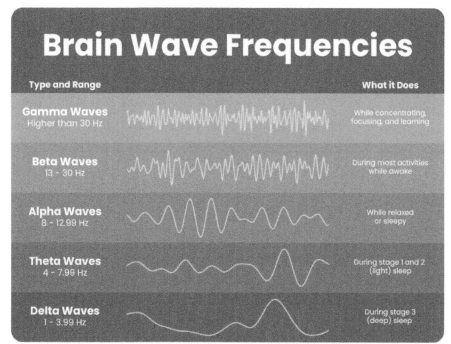

Our brain better computes the beat's frequency differences at lower volumes and shorter sessions, around five minutes.

Breathing

When you are stressed, you'll experience an increased rate of respiration, increased heart rate, and high blood pressure. When you take a deep breath, a message is sent to your brain to calm down and relax. The brain then transmits this message to your body, and your vitals (respiratory rate, heart rate, and blood pressure) all decrease as you breathe deeply to relax. This sequence makes your body feel like it does when you are already relaxed.

The way you breathe will affect your overall health. Breathing exercises are easy to learn. You can do them whenever you want, and you don't need any special tools or equipment to do them.

Take a minute when you first wake up, when you feel stressed, and before you go to sleep to practice some deep breathing exercises to decrease stress, relax your mind, increase healing, and improve sleep.

Belly Breathing Technique;

1. Sit or lie flat in a comfortable position.

2. Put one hand on your belly just below your ribs and the other hand on your chest.

3. Inhale slowly to the count of four through your nose (smell the roses), with abdomen expanding, relax, and listen to your breath. Your chest should not move.

4. Pause for one count.

5. Exhale slowly through pursed lips as if you were blowing out a candle to the count of six, with abdomen deflating, shoulders relaxed and engaged, listening to your breath. Feel the hand on your belly sink in, and use it to push all the air out.

6. Pause for one count.

7. Do this breathing 3 to 10 times. Take your time with each breath.

8. Notice how you feel at the end of the exercise.

9. Say or think calm when you inhale and smile when you exhale.

Some benefits of proper breathing;

- When you deep breathe, the body releases endorphins, which are natural pain killers and feel-good hormones.

- When we take deep breaths, the upward and downward movement of the diaphragm helps push blood through the body, increasing blood flow.

- Due to increased blood flow, we get more oxygen into

our blood, causing increased energy levels.

- Bad posture causes incorrect breathing. Rounded shoulders and a forward head posture causes the muscles around the chest to tighten, which inhibits the flow of air into your lungs. As you practice breathing exercises, your spine will straighten up, and allow more air into your lungs.

- Deep breathing reduces the acidity and stress in your body, making it alkaline. Reducing acidity will reduce inflammation in your body.

- Carbon dioxide is a natural toxic waste by-product of respiration. Improper breathing causes this waste to build up in your body, making it weaker and more susceptible to illness.

- Breathing correctly also helps lymph circulate more efficiently through the body. Improving lymph circulation will strengthen your immune system.

- The increased blood flow due to deep breathing also encourages intestinal action, which further improves your overall digestion. Also, deep breathing results in a calmer nervous system, which also improves digestion.

- When you are angry, anxious, or scared, your muscles tighten, and your breathing becomes shallow. Your breathing constricts, which causes decreased oxygen consumption. Long deep breathing reverses this process, allowing your body (and mind) to become calmer.

- There are many breathing techniques. Some breathing techniques include box, Wim Hof, ujjayi, the breath of fire, and alkaline breathing. Try out free tutorials on YouTube and see which you enjoy most.

Physical

When explaining musculoskeletal problems to patients, I

like to use the analogy of a spider web. When your muscles and bones are moving and functioning normally, your body is like a spider web where muscles, ligaments, tendons, and bones are anchored and pulling on one another with perfect balance so you can move fluidly and without pain or dysfunction.

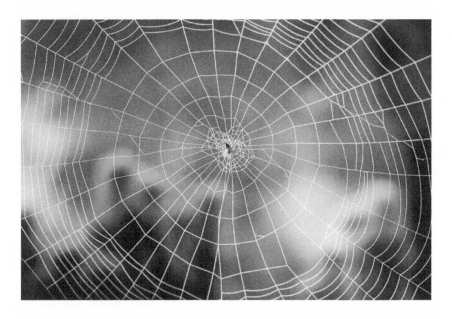

When a muscle, tendon, ligament, or bone is damaged, the others have to carry more load (weight) and do more work to compensate for the damaged one. The longer this imbalance exists, the more likely it is that you'll have additional damage to other body structures due to being overworked or simply being forced to work outside of their normal intended function. When this occurs, the spider web (muscles, tendons, ligaments, and bones) can become strained.

As you can see in the image below, the remaining strands of a spider web (analogous for muscles, tendons, ligaments, and bones) are resilient and doing what's necessary to keep the spider web (body) together. But it comes at a cost as significant deformity can occur in the spider web (body structure), due to overuse and changing the lines of pull.

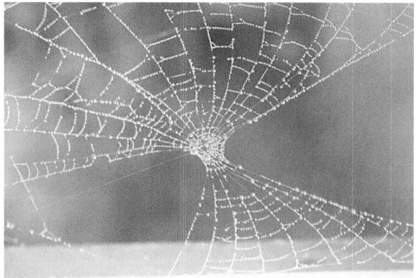

By observing and improving a person's biomechanics, we can correct some of the imbalances formed in your body due to injury.

One strategy used is called gait (walking) analysis, the systematic study of human motion, using the trained eye and the brain of observers, augmented by instrumentation for measuring body movements, body mechanics, and the activity of the muscles.

Gait analysis is used to correct or remediate disorders caused by abnormal walking patterns. Abnormal movement can translate into pain and deformity in almost any part of the body. By using a cane, braces, walker, splint, treatment, or crutches the abnormal gait can be improved, which translates to less pain and less dysfunction.

Another useful strategy is task analysis, where a person is observed performing a specific task, and recommendations are made to decrease discomfort for the person and make it easier for them to complete the task in the future. The components usually assessed include both manual and mental aspects of the task, task duration, and frequency. Specific recommendations are then made to correct your ergonomics (posture and movement during the task), so your body is not put under unnecessary stress by being in awkward postures, extreme temperature, or repeated movements that may hurt your musculoskeletal system.

Exercise

This is going to be one of the most important aspects of your recovery. Depending on your injury, exercise should start from day one, even if it's doing exercise in bed or just sitting up on the edge of the bed. In fact, research shows that even visualizing muscle contractions without actually exercising strengthen muscles by as much as 35 percent over a twelve-week period. When I sustained my most recent injury, I was exercising twice a day and preparing to compete in a wrestling meet. I was in tip-top condition, but after only a week of being in bed, I needed assistance just to sit at the edge of the bed. After a couple of weeks, I was able to build my strength to walk five steps to the toilet using crutches, but then I needed to stay on the toilet and rest for half an hour to build my strength back up to walk the five steps back to my bed where I would be exhausted for 2-3 hours. I was only able to complete this feat about once a day.

Being in bed causes;

- Loss of 1-3% of your strength per day and 10-20% per week.

- Rhabdomyolysis- a breakdown of damaged skeletal muscle.

- Muscle breakdown triggers the release of myoglobin, a protein that stores oxygen in your muscles. High amounts of myoglobin in your bloodstream can cause kidney damage.

- Contractures- a permanent shortening of a muscle or joint.

- Excretion of calcium as bone density decreases

- Heterotopic ossification- when the soft tissue surrounding a bone forms mature bone.

- Bedsores, also called pressure ulcers and decubitus ulcers, are skin sores that develop on the skin and underlying tissue as a result of prolonged pressure on the skin. Bedsores develop on skin that covers bony areas of the body such as, heels, ankles, hips, and tailbone.

- Endurance can be depleted at an even faster rate as your healing body utilizes all the calories, you're eating to prioritize healing.

- Lying in bed is also associated with an increased risk of stress, depression, and several other psychological and cardiovascular ailments.

We don't think about it much, but just working on your activities of daily living; working, gardening, cleaning, and self-care requires a certain amount of daily strength and endurance. As you stop completing even these basic activities your body begins to lose strength and endurance quickly.

Exercise; work with your rehabilitation team (doctor and therapists) to put together a comprehensive workout plan for your rehabilitation. Be consistent and don't skip on your rehabilitation. You could end up with lifelong problems if you don't put in the time now to properly rehabilitate yourself. Whether you're a professional athlete or an ordinary person, lost time is lost productivity, so the faster you can get back to your activities of daily living, the faster your life is going to be back to normal. Most patients I see have families or households to support and can't afford to sit around and heal slowly.

Be patient, it's common that I'll see a person in the hospital for one injury and once they're discharged, they come back with another broken bone because they tried to do too much and fell and broke something else.

My Exercise Strategies

Get a calendar and write down what activities you have scheduled for which days. Pick your favorite music to workout to. People workout longer and more vigorously to music. A comprehensive exercise program works your entire body, not just the affected area. Mostly because the weaker or injured body part is going to need support from the rest of your body. Therefore, strengthening your entire body is going to help the injured area heal faster. Aside from your targeted exercises, engage in whole-body workouts such as swimming or walking as your injury allows.

Bed Exercises

Start immediately with bed exercises. Physical activity increases blood flow throughout the body, which can keep bed sores from developing and improve overall health.

1. Palm stretch

With an open palm, extend your fingers as much as you can with pressure for a few seconds. Then, touch your thumb with each finger. Repeat this exercise a couple of times on each hand every day.

2. Ankle plantarflexion-dorsiflexion exercise

As you're lying on your back, ask your caregiver to hold one ankle and heel and bend the foot forward for several seconds. Then, ask your caretaker to push your foot upward.

3. Arm lift

Lift your arm as high as you can and hold it there for 10 seconds. Repeat on the other arm. If you're unable to hold your arm up for that long, place your upper arm on the bed and bend your elbow until it reaches a 90-degree angle.

4. Leg lift

While lying on your back, keep your leg straight while lifting it up and toward the ceiling. Hold it there for 10 to 20 seconds, then bring the leg down. Alternate the same exercise on the other leg.

Completing these exercises a few times a day will help prevent some of the negative consequences of being in bed.

Stretching

As we age, we lose 10% of our flexibility per decade. Movement of the joint and the stress of movement helps keep the fluid moving in the joints. Being inactive causes the cartilage to shrink and stiffen, reducing joint mobility. Once you're able to get out of bed, you can start a daily stretch regime to help maintain joint mobility.

Yoga is an excellent option to use for its strengthening and simultaneous stretching components. Below is a sample yoga program for beginners for enhancing and maintaining mobility after an injury. Assuming each position for thirty seconds, each will allow you to complete a stretch routine in 3-5 minutes.

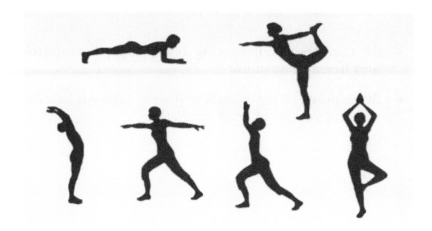

Swimming

Once your wounds close up start swimming three days a

week every other day. Do not swim with open wounds. Chlorinated or salt pool water can slow the healing process and cause irritation, and bacteria in the water will increase the risk of your wound becoming infected. A wound that is healing should remain dry.

If your mobility is limited use a pool that is handicap accessible. A pool lift allows you to transfer from a sitting position into a pool and lift you out again when you're done swimming.

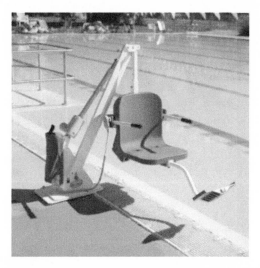

- 30 minutes of alternating backstroke, breaststroke, and freestyle swimming

- 30 minutes of aqua jogging (Use a flotation belt early on until you build your strength).

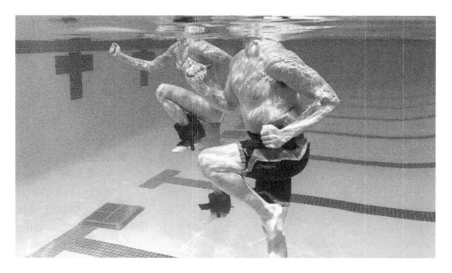

- 30-60 minutes of walking, running, and leg exercises see routine below.

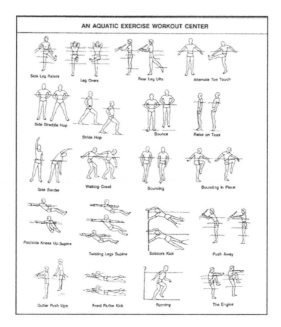

Weight Training

Initially, I could only exercise with resistance bands, then as I built my strength, I started lifting weights. During the time I was in a wheelchair, I only did leg exercises with resistance bands and pool exercises. Free weights were only used for my upper body and slowly introduced to my lower body as my bones healed. Weightlift on the three days that you're not swimming and rest on the seventh day of the week.

One of the most effective exercise techniques you can use is **Peripheral Heart Action (PHA) Workouts.** You alternate one upper body exercise with one lower body exercise to force your heart to pump blood to the extreme ends of the body so blood doesn't localize. You can create your own PHA workout using anything from resistance bands and dumbbells, to barbells and kettlebells.

For beginners, this type of workout will be more intense than a typical circuit training workout. Start out with lighter weights, fewer circuits, and simpler exercises until you get used to it.

To make your own PHA workout:

Pick six exercises, three for the lower body, and three for the upper body. You can pick compound exercises to add intensity. For example, pushups, squats, dumbbell rows, lunges, biceps curls, and leg lifts.

- Start with enough weight so you tire at 8-10 reps. To begin, use little or no weight and slowly work your way up to heavier weights.

- Alternate an upper and a lower body exercise with no rest in between.

- After the first circuit, rest for a minute and then complete one to six cycles as you advance.

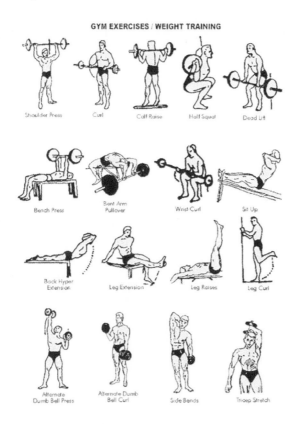

GYM EXERCISES / WEIGHT TRAINING

Treatments

Collaborate with all of your medical team including your acupressurist, massage therapist, occupational therapist, physical therapist, or any other type of practitioner to make sure that they're updating your treatment plan as needed.

Shaolin Medical Treatments

Shaolin Chan Medicine can be traced to the Shaolin Temple in China. It is a monastery where monks practice martial arts, meditate, and practice Shaolin. The philosophy of Shaolin includes energy, healing, physical conditioning, control, balance, flexibility, speed, agility, and power. Over time the monks began to accumulate medical experience by taking advantage of abundant herbal resources in the Song Mountain and benefitting from the folk medical approaches. They developed Qigong therapy, massage therapy and pointing therapy which is used for medical treatments. Shaolin Medicine can treat various diseases, treat traumatic injuries, and has many divisions such as surgery and internal departments.

I started with three visits a week and tapered down visits as I made progress during my recovery.

Acupuncture

An acupuncturist inserts hair-thin needles at specific body points or energy pathways to restore the flow of qi. The needles stimulate acupoints, which cause the nervous system to release opium-like endorphins to the muscles, spinal cord, and brain. These chemicals reduce the pain experience and trigger the release of other chemicals and hormones that influence the body's internal regulating system. Research shows that acupuncture promotes complete bone healing, improved range of motion, and facilitates faster reductions in swelling and pain.

Throughout the years, I've tried just about every treatment I was taught on reducing swelling, and in my experience, I've never found anything as effective as acupuncture. I've had some terrible injuries and seen patients with some that I thought would stay swollen for weeks. After only one treatment with acupuncture, I've observed swelling reduce in one day, to where you couldn't even tell there was an injury. Depending on your injury, it's recommended you start with three visits a week and taper down visits as you make progress during your recovery.

Bone Stimulator

The Bone stimulator is a machine that emits a pulsed electromagnetic or ultrasonic impulse to the area where bone healing should occur. The machine is worn for an amount of time prescribed by your physician, usually 1-2 hours a day for 3-9 months. The bone stimulator activates a series of receptors in the body to facilitate the healing response. Essentially, the bone stimulator creates a low-level electrical field which activates molecular signaling pathways, increases the number of bone cells, and increases bone strength and quality. I used a bone stimulator every day for nine months.

Hyperbaric Chamber

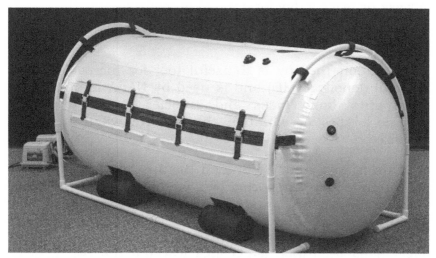

Hyperbaric oxygen therapy (HBOT) accelerates the healing process of almost any medical disorder.

You enter a chamber with pressure levels of 1.5 to 3 times higher than average, relax, sit, or lie comfortably and breathe in pure oxygen using a mask. Oxygen is forced into the blood, infusing the injured tissues that need more oxygen so that they can begin healing and restore healthy body function.

HBOT prevents "reperfusion injury," which is tissue damage that happens when blood supply returns to tissues after being deprived of oxygen. Damaged cells start releasing harmful free radicals into the body. Free radicals damage body tissues, cause the blood vessels to clamp up, and stop blood flow. HBOT helps the body's oxygen radical scavengers to find the problem molecules and assist healing to continue.

HBOT helps block harmful bacteria from releasing toxins into the body and strengthens the body's immune system. It also increases the concentration of oxygen in the tissues, which fight infections, and helps white blood cells find and destroy invaders.

HBOT promotes the formation of new collagen, blood vessels, and skin cells. It also stimulates cells to produce vascular endothelial growth factor, which attracts and stimulates endothelial cells necessary for healing.

For faster results HBOT can be used at least three times a week or twice a day for optimal outcomes.

Vibration Therapy

Vibration therapy is a useful tool for increasing bone mineral density (BMD) and is used by NASA to strengthen astronauts' bone mass and muscles. The two most common types of vibration therapy are whole-body and localized.

During whole-body vibration therapy, you stand, sit, or lay on a machine supported by a vibrating platform. Whole-body treatment will work out your entire body and is best when you have at least weight-bearing as tolerated status for your bone fracture. It can be used for upper or lower body bone fractures, while also working the rest of your body. A typical exercise may include standing in a half-squat position with your knees bent.

During localized vibration therapy, a hand-held vibrating device is placed on a specific part of the body for targeted treatments. As the vibrations transmit through the body, they cause the muscles to contract and relax, which causes muscle strengthening. Vibrations also stimulate the body to produce more osteoblasts (build bone), stimulate bone formation, and improve bone strength.

Vibration machines produce vertical, up and down, front and back, and sideways vibrations. Up and down waves are the most effective for producing rapid muscle contractions. The intensity of vibrations will affect the efficacy of the treatment.

Circulating Cold Water Therapy System

After surgery you're going to need to ice your surgical site to decrease swelling. Applying bags of ice or frozen peas is an option, however, the condensation from the ice bags wets your bedding and only lasts for short periods of time before you have to replace the melted ice. An ice circulating machine is one of the best devices I've come across for drug-free pain relief and edema management after an injury or post-surgery. The machine is extremely easy-to-use and can be used for knees, shoulders, back, hips, ankles, elbows, calves, limbs, and any other part of your body necessary. It's a very effective strategy to avoid using pain medications.

Low-Level Laser Therapy

Low-level light therapy (LLLT) is a more intense version of near-infrared (NIR) light. It is a cold laser that concentrates light on one area of your body. Low-power laser application will relieve pain, promote healing, and enhance cell function. In clinical studies, LLLT increases strength, speeds up muscle recovery and healing post-surgery, decreases inflammation, and reduces chronic and acute pain. LLLT stimulates mitochondria to boost ATP production resulting in increased energy and blood flow, facilitating the fracture-repair process through several mechanisms that accelerate callus formation.

Near-Infrared Light (NIR) Therapy

Near-infrared light (NIR) therapy is a proven way to immediately increase ATP production by osteoblasts and fibroblasts in the process of bone healing. Infrared light is a specific wavelength of light that donates photons to your mitochondria via molecules called cytochromes, promoting cell repair, decreasing pain and inflammation, promoting weight loss, and enhancing the healing process. Its ability to penetrate deep down into the skin allows it to reach the cells' mitochondria, also known as the cell's power plants, and stimulate them to increase adenosine triphosphate (ATP) production. Resulting in recharging of your mitochondria, stimulation of DNA and RNA synthesis, increased blood flow, which activates the lymphatic system, resulting in increased waste removal and tissue repair. Increased ATP provides you with steady energy all day and better sleep at night. Red light also triggers collagen synthesis, and collagen represents more than 90% of the organic bone matrix. More collagen also means younger-looking skin and faster wound healing.

Different hues of light have various therapeutic effects on the body. Red light stimulates melatonin production, which will help you improve your sleep and promote recovery during sleep. If used a few minutes before physical exercise, red and infrared light can boost strength and prevent soreness. Wavelengths of red and infrared light 660 to 905 nanometers reach skeletal muscle tissue, stimulating the mitochondria to produce more ATP, which cells use as fuel.

Although excessive exposure to blue light from electronics at night can be detrimental, exposure to blue light during the day can improve reaction time, alertness, focus, and productivity. High amounts of bright daylight hitting photoreceptors in the eye will suppress melatonin levels and set off receptors in the brain that energize you. Stand or sit by windows or go outside as much as possible every day to increase your dosage of blue rays from natural light.

Greenlight can reduce chronic pain caused by migraines or fibromyalgia by up to 60 percent. Greenlight increases the production of pain-killing opioid-like chemicals called enkephalins. Enkephalins reduce inflammation, which plays a role in many chronic pain conditions. One to two hours of green light a day can decrease migraines and other types of chronic pain.

Massage

Massage therapy helps relax muscle tissue, decrease

nerve compression, increase joint space, increase range of motion, improve circulation, and has a calming effect. I tried to get a massage daily if possible, from family, friends, or sometimes going to a professional. Massage helps nutrients and oxygen to flow into swollen and damaged areas to help expedite healing.

Grounding

Grounding, also known as earthing, is the process of transferring the Earth's electrons into the body from walking barefoot outside, sitting, working, or sleeping indoors connected to conductive systems that transfer the Earth's electrons from the ground into the body. The Earth contains free electrons, which can reach the body when it is in direct contact with the ground. The electrons act as antioxidants to neutralize compounds known as reactive oxygen species, which can damage the cells in excess. The process causes the development of antioxidants, better sleep, and reduced pain.

When I could not walk, I would sit barefoot with my feet resting on the dirt. As my mobility improved, I would walk either with crutches or unsupported on the soil barefoot so my body could absorb free electrons from the Earth.

Sun Bathing

Natural sunlight hitting the skin triggers the body's production of vitamin D. Vitamin D is a hormone produced by the kidneys that control blood calcium concentration and helps the immune system. Without Vitamin D, our bodies cannot effectively absorb calcium, which is essential to building strong bones and muscles.

Vitamin D is also known as calcitriol, ergocalciferol, calcidiol, and cholecalciferol. Vitamin D is produced by the body when sunlight hits the skin causing a chemical reaction that produces it. It is an important hormone that protects against inflammation, builds muscle, lowers high blood pressure, protects against cancer, and improves brain function.

Regular sun exposure is needed to maintain healthy blood levels of vitamin D, 10–30 minutes of midday sunlight, several times per week. People with darker skin have more melanin, which works as a natural sunblock against sunlight, therefore they require more sun exposure to get the needed vitamin D.

Diet

If you don't give your body what it needs to heal, it will find a way to leech what it needs from other bones or tissues in your body which will make you weaker, slow your healing, and increase your risk for other bone injuries, infections, and health problems.

Avoid foods that drain minerals from your body such as; caffeine, nightshade vegetables, spinach, alcohol, sugar, and fruit juices. Also, avoid foods that you may be allergic to such as wheat (gluten) or peanuts. Try to eat as much home-prepared food as possible, as the less processed the food the more nutrient-dense it tends to be.

My diet consisted of as much home-cooked food as possible. In the beginning, while I had open wounds that were healing, I ate;

- One whole head of raw garlic a day mashed up and eaten raw with other foods throughout the day. Garlic is antimicrobial, antiviral, and antiparasitic, so it helps prevent infections. Garlic has also been shown to minimize bone loss by increasing estrogen in females. Garlic and onions are also beneficial for diminishing the effects of osteoarthritis.

- 16-24 glasses of water with lemon juice a day. The fresh lemon juice gave me vitamin C for wound healing and helped purge my liver of toxins from the medications I was taking.

- Ovo-lacto Vegetarian (eggs, dairy, fruits, and vegetables). Digesting meat is work and you want your body working on healing your bones instead of digesting meat.

- Half a teaspoon of turmeric, Ceylon cinnamon, and ginger three times a day. All three are effective anti-inflammatories.

- 1 liter of plain Kefir yogurt a day without added sugar. Kefir is high in protein, easy to digest since the lactose is digested by the bacteria, and contains 12 different types of bacteria in it.

- Half a pineapple every day until completely healed. Pineapples are rich in vitamins and antioxidants which boost the immune system, build strong bones, aid indigestion, and reduce bruising and pain that occurs after surgery. Pineapples also have enzymes including bromelain which helps to reduce swelling and inflammation. Eating pineapples can reduce your recovery time from surgery.

- One teaspoon of Medium-chain triglyceride (MCT) oil before going to sleep.

- Coconut oil for cooking. Coconut oil has a higher smoke point than most other vegetable oils, so it doesn't oxidize and cause damage to you. Coconut oil is high in healthy saturated fats that can boost fat burning, provide your body and brain with quick energy, raise the good HDL cholesterol in your blood, and reduces heart disease.

- Collagen protein or homemade protein powder for shakes when I wasn't hungry, but knew I needed more calories as I was 20% below my typical weight.

- Bone broth for extra minerals necessary for bone reconstruction.

- Gelatin for large doses of collagen which breaks down into amino acids for bone reconstruction.

Medication

Fill prescriptions as needed and prescribed to help you deal with many of the symptoms common when a bone injury is sustained. Allowing symptoms such as pain, inflammation, nausea, loss of appetite, or other negative symptoms can slow your progress and lead to unnecessary delays in your recovery. Inversely as your pain decreases, swelling subsides, and other symptoms start to fade work with your medical team to cut back on medications as soon as possible. Although medications have many health benefits, they also come with many side effects which can cause unnecessary stress on your body and even slow your healing.

Consult with your naturopathic doctor or other healthcare professional to adjust your herbal regime throughout your healing process. As with any medication you have to ensure there is a fit between what your taking and what is needed at each stage of your recovery.

Supplements

Due to over-farming and soil erosion, most farmers are experiencing soil depletion of minerals. This causes fruits and vegetables farmed on depleted soil to lack or have lower quantities of essential minerals. This translates to lower nutritional content for some fruits and vegetables. For this reason, it's important to supplement your diet with vitamins and minerals.

Your body only needs a small number of vitamins and minerals every day. A varied diet generally provides enough of each vitamin and mineral, however, some people may need supplements to correct deficiencies, and their bone injury may require particular vitamins or minerals.

For example, let's say you eat some broccoli. Your body benefits from everything in the broccoli, but your bones may specifically need extra boron which is not an easy mineral to get in your diet. So, by eating more broccoli, your body can extract more boron from the broccoli. Whatever excess vitamin C, calcium, or other nutrients that are in the broccoli that your body does not need will be excreted out of your body harmlessly. By eating the extra broccoli, you gain access to the extra reserves of boron. In most fruits and vegetables there are always going to be some nutrients that are more abundant than others. In general, most minerals, are only available in low concentrations in food. I'd like to think of them as the rare earth metals of the body.

In our natural world, there are lots of metals that are abundant such as aluminum, copper, lead, etc. But then there are the rare earth metals that are also readily available but only in very low quantities so you have to mine and refine tons and tons of dirt just to come up with ounces of the metal that we need to make iPhones, missiles, electric cars, satellites, computers, and other high tech devices.

Minerals are the same way in food. They are present in very low quantities in the foods you eat, so eating a variety of foods on a regularly will get you the nutrition your body needs, except when you have a traumatic injury that requires major reconstruction such as broken bones. Having broken bones is going to require that you make dramatic nutritional changes to support the new bone growth and reconstruction. Not doing so will delay the process or give you unfavorable outcomes such as a delayed healing response, bone deformities, or collateral damage due to inflammation. Although inflammation is beneficial, it can also slow bone reconstruction. The inflammatory process can cause a bottleneck in the circulatory system so that oxygen, nutrients, and the immune system are not able to respond as quickly as possible. In some situations, taking anti-inflammatory medications can be even worse.

Non-steroidal, anti-inflammatory drugs (NSAIDs) are commonly prescribed to reduce inflammation and promote healing. The theory is that if we reduce the swelling, it'll speed healing. The problem with that theory is that the inflammatory response is one of the body's natural responses to increase healing. Reducing inflammation too quickly, will slow the healing process.

By eating food that naturally fights inflammation, your body will have to invest less energy to do so and instead use its power for healing.

Consider weightlifting, you lift weights to make your muscles bigger so that you can have a beach body. Adding extra protein in your diet will help facilitate that process of making your muscles bigger, faster. Therefore, eating the protein will help you reach your goal of having bigger more defined muscles.

In the case of bones, your outcomes are not usually visible so you have to do the same thing but without the visual feedback or markers that you would normally have when building muscle. This is one of the core reasons that rebuilding bone can be a challenge.

Supplement Regime

When taking supplements (day and night) or eating foods containing fat-soluble vitamins such as vitamins A, E, D, and K (foods like carrots, leafy green veggies, and legumes), pair them with a dietary fat such as olive oil, fish oil, coconut oil, or butter (In moderation). Dietary fats significantly increase the body's ability for nutrient absorption. An example would be having a salad with an olive oil-based dressing or taking your fish oil, krill oil, astaxanthin, or MCT coconut oil with your supplements.

Some supplements are better absorbed and used by your body when taken at different times of the day. See chapter 22 for dosage;

For accelerated fat loss and muscle building, drink "Hardcore Juice" as your first meal.

Hardcore Juice:

Use a Vitamix 64-ounce blender to blend the ingredients below and refrigerate in glass bottles.

1 teaspoon of MCT Oil (Fat burning Brain Booster)

1 tablespoon of Turmeric Powder (Anti-inflammatory, stabilizes blood sugar, good for heart, brain, and bones)

1/2 teaspoon of Ceylon Cinnamon (Anti-inflammatory, stabilizes blood sugar, good for heart, brain, and bones)

1 tablespoon of Cocoa Powder (Anti-inflammatory, stabilizes blood sugar, good for heart, brain, and bones)

1 teaspoon of pure Vanilla extract (Antioxidant, anticancer, anti-inflammatory, neuroprotective)

1 teaspoon Creatine Monohydrate Powder (Improve strength, increase lean muscle mass, and speed recovery after exercise)

1/2 teaspoon HMB Powder (Improve strength, increase lean muscle mass, and speed recovery after exercise, especially in older adults)

1/2 teaspoon Beta-Alanine (Increased exercise capacity, decreases muscle fatigue, antioxidant with immune-enhancing and anti-aging properties)

1 teaspoon Glutamine (Boosts immune system, rebuilds intestinal health, benefits leaky gut, spurs muscle growth and running speed, reduces sugar and carb cravings)

1 1/4 teaspoon L-Citrulline DL-Malate 2:1 (Increased nitric oxide production, enhanced endurance and exercise performance, reduced muscle soreness, support for cardiovascular health, ammonia clearance, and potential erectile function support)

1 teaspoon of Beet Powder (Improved athletic performance, reduced blood pressure, improved brain function, lowered risk of cancer, enhanced cardiovascular health, increased endurance and reduced fatigue, antioxidant properties, support for liver health, digestive health)

1 1/2 teaspoon Acacia Fiber (Lowers bad cholesterol levels, keeps blood sugar in check, prevents diabetes, and helps treat irritable bowel syndrome (IBS))

1 teaspoon of Bee Pollen (Anti-inflammatory, improved immunity, menopausal symptoms, and wound healing.)

1/2 teaspoon pf Royal Jelly (Anti-inflammatory, improved immunity, antioxidant properties, improved cognitive function, anti-tumor, blood sugar control, balances hormones, decreases cholesterol, and protects liver.)

4 tablespoons of collagen peptides (18 grams of protein) (Improve digestion, strengthen joints and bones, improve the health of hair, skin, nails, and cognitive function)

1 teaspoon Matcha Green Tea powder (Powerful antioxidant, increases cognitive function, cleans the liver, prevents cancer, weight loss, and improves cardiovascular health)

Optional add vegan protein powder, Greek yogurt, kefir, and/or high protein soy milk. If you're using vegan protein powder, add 20% more to account for decreased bioavailability. Use 1/2 gram of protein powder for every pound of body weight. For example, I weigh 200 lbs, so I consume 100 grams daily. I would add half of my daily protein requirement, 50 grams, to my Hardcore Juice.

Mix in 20 ounces of warm water (not from a plastic bottle) or warm soy milk for 30-60 seconds (mixing time is essential to promote the creation of EZ water).

health goals.

Use your Hardcore Juice to take your morning supplements.

1. Calcium (1000-1200 mg as calcium carbonate)

Most vegetarians are deficient in calcium. Calcium builds and maintains strong bones. The heart, muscles, and nerves also need calcium to function properly. 7/10 people are deficient.

2. Nicotinamide mononucleotide (NMN) (1g)

NMN has been able to suppress age-associated weight gain, enhance energy metabolism and physical activity, improve insulin sensitivity, improve eye function, improve mitochondrial metabolism and prevent age-linked changes in gene expression.

3. Resveratrol (1g)

Resveratrol has antioxidant and anti-inflammatory properties to protect you against diseases like cancer, diabetes, and Alzheimer's disease. The anti-inflammatory effects of resveratrol make it a good remedy for arthritis and skin inflammation.

4. Potato Starch (1 tablespoon) Helps to control hunger, improve digestion, and immune health, control blood sugar, and manage weight. (To be used if you're still feeling hungry when going out to eat or to a party.) Potato starch is also prebiotic, feeding beneficial gut bacteria. The fermentation of resistant starch in the colon produces short-chain fatty acids like butyrate, which is helpful for colon health and a healthy gut microbiome.

Brain boosting Supplements (generally one hour before starting work activities)

1. Citicoline (500–2,000 mg) Improves cognition and prevents cognitive decline

2. Theacrine (50 to 300 mg) Increases energy and improves cognitive function

3. Pyrroloquinoline Quinone (PQQ) (20mg) Raises blood flow to the cerebral cortex, improving attention, thinking, and memory.

4. L-Theanine (100-400 mg) Improves cognitive function, eases anxiety, stress, and reduces insomnia.

5. Genius Mushrooms. A type of fungi that increases blood flow and oxygen levels to the brain, which improves memory and cognitive function.

Relaxation (taken in the morning to help promote a peaceful day)

1. Bach Rescue Remedy (1 drop a day) Used to relieve anxiety, nervous tension, stress, agitation or despair and provide a sense of focus and calm.

MORNING Supplements (Taken with the first meal to

increase absorption and boost performance for the day)

1. Metformin (500 mg) (prescription) In 1918, scientists discovered that the medicinal herb French Lilac (Galega officinalis) contained guanidine, which could lower blood sugar. Medicines containing guanidine, such as Metformin, were developed to treat diabetes. In 1995, the FDA approved Metformin for the treatment of diabetes. Since then, it has become the most widely prescribed medication for diabetes. Metformin is approved for the treatment of type 2 diabetes. However, it is also used off-label to treat polycystic ovarian syndrome (PCOS), infertility, weight reduction, diabetes prevention, pregnancy complications, and obesity. Recent Harvard studies suggest that Metformin may increase life expectancy by an average of ten years and slow aging by improving the body's responsiveness to insulin, antioxidant effects, and blood vessel health. Activated Protein Kinase (AMPK metabolic activator) (450 mg) is a non-prescription less effective alternative.

Some studies have suggested that metformin may positively affect bone metabolism. Bone metabolism ensures the body's maintenance of bone strength and mineral homeostasis.

2. Multivitamin with Iron. Vegetarians often do not get 8-18mg of iron daily. A multivitamin covers many supplements (iron, b-vitamins, copper, zinc) so you can cut down on the number of pills you take and replace the need to take a b-complex if you decide to cut back.

3. Vitamin A (3000-10,000 IU as retinyl palmitate) If you aren't consuming organ meats such as beef kidney, liver, or heart, then you're not going to get sufficient amounts of vitamin A in your diet. You can't get vitamin A from plants, and vegetables such as carrots won't help because they have beta-carotene instead of vitamin A. Vegetarians should take vitamin A because beta-carotene is poorly converted into vitamin A. Half of the population is deficient in this vitamin.

Don't take vitamin A supplements without consulting with a doctor if you have kidney disease, liver disease, or drink heavily.

4. Vitamin B-complex. Vitamin B-complex is a must for people like myself who eat a vegan and vegetarian plant-based diet which is typically deficient in B-vitamins. Vitamin B-complex relieves stress, boosts cognitive performance, and reduces symptoms of depression and anxiety.

5. Vitamin C (500-1000 mg as Ascorbic acid or liposomal) Vitamin C is the safest supplement you can take. It is used for collagen and connective tissue formation, making glutathione, the most potent antioxidant in the body, and preventing free radical damage. Vitamin C is heat-sensitive, so heating vegetables and fruits will destroy it. Take higher doses of vitamin C when you're sick. Half of the population is deficient.

6. Vitamin D (1,000 mg per 25 lbs of body weight) Vitamin D helps regulate the amount of calcium and phosphate in the body needed to keep bones, teeth and muscles healthy. Because most of us work indoors, most people are deficient. Up to 9/10 people are deficient in this vitamin.

7. Vitamin E (400 IU as D-Alpha-Tocopherol) Naturally sourced vitamin E is called d-alpha-tocopherol and is the preferred form of vitamin E transported and used by the liver. The synthetically produced form is labeled as dl-alpha-tocopherol and made from petroleum products.

The RDA for vitamin E is 15 mg, but the upper tolerable intake level (UL) for vitamin E is 1,000 mg (1,500 IU). Research shows the optimal dose for disease prevention and treatment for adults is 400 to 800 IU per day. 8/10 people are deficient.

8. Vitamin K2 (100 mcg) It's difficult to get enough of this vitamin in your daily diet. Vitamin K2 activates a protein that helps calcium bind to bones, improving bone density and reducing the risk of bone fractures.

9. Probiotic (10 to 20 billion colony-forming units (CFU) Probiotics provide a wide variety of benefits against a range of health conditions, including allergies, arthritis, asthma, cancer, mental issues, and digestive problems. I take it to help keep my microbiome healthy.

10. Astaxanthin (10mg) Protects cells from damage, improves immune functions, athletic performance, aging skin, and reduces muscle soreness from exercise. It also helps with the absorption of fat-soluble vitamins.

11. Pycnogenol (pine bark, 400mg) Improves circulation, lowers blood pressure, and has anti-aging benefits.

12. Coenzyme Q10 (CoQ10) (300mg) It improves heart health, regulates blood sugar, assists in preventing and treating cancer, reduces the frequency of migraines, and reduces the oxidative damage that leads to muscle fatigue, skin damage, and brain and lung diseases.

13. Chlorella (5 grams) A good source of several vitamins, minerals, and antioxidants, it detoxifies the body and improves cholesterol and blood sugar levels.

14. Odorless Garlic Extract (1200mg) Lowers blood pressure, improves circulation, is an antioxidant, and contains neuroprotection properties.

15. Epigallocatechin Gallate (EGCG) (400 mg) Green tea extract, reduces inflammation, promotes weight loss, and helps prevent heart and brain disease.

16. Silicea (9-14 mg) Promotes collagen production, the body's most abundant protein, helps rebuild bones, skin, and joints.

17. Sea Kelp (500 mcg Iodine supplement) High in minerals and antioxidants, boosts energy, and improves muscle recovery.

18. Ashwagandha (1000 mg) is an adaptogenic herb clinically shown to help reduce stress, regulate cortisol levels, enhance focus, memory, and mental stamina, and reduce irritability and stress-related cravings. Improves sleep, lowers blood glucose levels and triglycerides, improves sexual function in women, supports heart health increases VO2 max levels, which is the maximum amount of oxygen you take in during physical exertion. Recent studies show that ashwagandha can increase testosterone levels in men by 10-15%, increasing strength and muscle size in men and not female participants.

NIGHT (Take with your last meal)

1. Metformin (2nd dose a day as needed) (500 mg) (prescription) Reduces fat storage, increases insulin sensitivity (to lower blood glucose), reduces cholesterol/triglyceride production, suppresses chronic inflammation, anti-aging, and increases lifespan.

2. Dehydroepiandrosterone (DHEA) (100mg) Improves cognitive function, erectile function, and helps prevent obesity.

3. L-Arginine (1-2 grams) & L-Ornithine (500-1000mg) (1 pill best taken together) Lowers blood pressure (if you take a blood pressure medication talk to your doctor before using it,) and treats erectile dysfunction. L-ornithine reduces fatigue and improves measures of athletic performance such as speed, strength, and power. Taking L-ornithine in combination with L-arginine also enhances strength and power in weightlifters.

4. Alpha-Lipoic Acid (225mg) & Acetyl L-Carnitine (525mg) (Combined in 1 pill) Alpha-lipoic acid is a potent antioxidant that reduces inflammation and skin aging, improves nerve function, lowers heart disease risk factors, and slows memory loss disorders.) Acetyl l-carnitine boosts your brain, mood, endurance, memory, strength and helps your body burn fat and recover from a workout.

5. Gamma-Aminobutyric Acid (GABA) (750mg) Improves mood, relieves anxiety, and improves sleep.

6. Glutamine (1000mg) Speeds muscle recovery and promotes muscle growth.

7. Magnesium Glycinate (400 mg) Essential for maintaining good health and plays a crucial role in everything from exercise performance to heart health and brain function. 50% of people are deficient.

8. Glutathione (1000mg) Promotes tissue building and repair, and immune system function.

9. Hyaluronic Acid (100 mg) Alleviates dry skin, reduces the appearance of fine lines and wrinkles and speeds up wound healing.

10. Krill Oil (500 mg) An excellent alternative to fish oil which often has contaminants and spoils quickly. Krill oil is high in omega-3 fatty acids that improve heart health, fight inflammation, and support brain and nervous system health.

11. Melatonin as needed (5mg) According to the National Institute of Health {NIH), Melatonin is the primary hormone regulating our sleep-wake cycle, the circadian rhythm. It is found in high concentrations in the mitochondria and is a mitochondria-targeted antioxidant, which indicates that it is an anti-aging mechanism. Melatonin is the most effective lipophilic antioxidant, proven twice as effective as vitamin E at preventing oxidative stress and cellular apoptosis.

Social

Social support after an injury is one of the most important and often overlooked factors in facilitating recovery from injury. After an injury, your social and physical needs for assistance are going to increase significantly. Especially if you are non-weight bearing or bed bound.

After an injury, the first thing that comes into question for most people is their self-efficacy. This reflects the person's confidence in their ability to exert control over one's own motivation, behavior, and social environment. You may start to question your abilities and it's normal to have self-doubt. Having and building a strong support group during recovery is important in helping you heal faster and support your psychological and physical needs.

Being injured will remove you from your typical routine, so you may lose contact with those you see everyday, or be forced to spend long periods of time isolated at home in bed. This adjustment can be difficult and it's normal to feel lonely. However, allowing these feelings to linger and not addressing the fundamental issues of isolation can cause regression in your rehabilitation. Consider making contact with old friends and family, hosting dinners, using a wheelchair to go out in public, and trying to follow as normal a social routine as possible. Humans need social interactions, the lack of such connections can lead to many problems, including depression and loneliness.

Spending large amounts of time in internet communities can decrease your interpersonal skills, increase anxiety, increase isolation, and cause depression. There's no replacement for face to face interactions and the multiple health benefits it provides.

Friends and family can also help run errands, complete household chores, and help fill in wherever you're in need. Additionally, keeping your spirits up is an objective measure that is difficult to measure, but has a profound impact on someone's recovery.

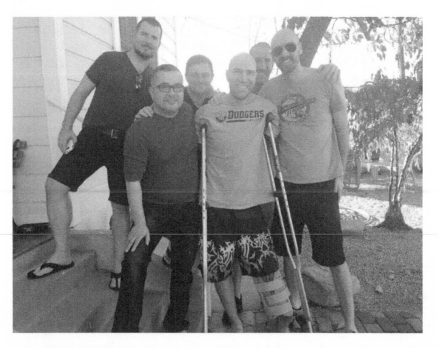

Spiritual

Spirituality is that part of you that helps you find meaning, connectedness, and purpose in your life. Spirituality generally leads to better health outcomes.

Spirituality helps people to cope with illness, suffering, recovery, and death. Spiritual health is achieved when you feel at peace with your life. Balancing the spiritual aspects of your life will lead to better physical healing. Whatever religion you practice, take some time to reflect and practice your faith.

There is an established link between connectedness factors, including religion, spirituality, social support, social participation, and health. Research has shown an improvement in the immune response to illness, stabilization of hormonal response, decreased anxiety, reduced inflammation, improved mood, increased benefit from vaccines, and the increase in feelings of happiness.

One of the best ways to make yourself and others happy is to give of yourself to others. By committing random acts of kindness, community service, and giving to others, you connect with a more abundant energy source that enhances your own. Assisting others is one of the most rewarding, healing, energy-producing activities you can do, and it's been shown to increase healing and reduce depression.

Mental

Besides your other needs, mental health is one of the most important for controlling stress and stressors. Various forms of meditation can be used to build mental health, including mindfulness meditation, repeating a mantra, guided imagery, or visualization. By reducing the sympathetic nervous system's anxiety-inducing fight or flight response, meditation can decrease your heart rate, lower your blood pressure, relax your muscles, and slow your breathing. Meditation also structurally changes the brain's cerebral cortex, which plays an instrumental role in memory, attention, and consciousness. Meditation can treat anxiety, stress, chronic pain, depression, and cancer. The psychological benefits include increased emotional stability, calmness, decreased anxiety, and greater self-confidence.

Emotional

When you feel good about yourself, it's much easier to cope with the ups and downs of life. Keep in mind during your healing process that this may be one of the only opportunities you have to spend days, weeks, or months to do as you like, free from having to go to work, and some of the other responsibilities you may have. People tend to give you some slack when you're injured and healing. Enjoy the time off, and take the opportunity to do something you've always wanted to do. With your new-found wealth of free time, you can; learn a language, create art, learn how to play an instrument, travel, or catch up with old friends and family. Make this one of your most memorable times in your life, instead of the opposite. I used my nine months off from work to visit friends, have gatherings with family and friends at my place, and travel. Although I was low on funds, I knew I was going to be returning to work sooner or later, so I took some zero interest 18-month loans out on my credit cards to travel, and then paid them back when I went back to work. Reframe things, change your perspective. Solve the solvable and leave the rest behind.

Ten Strategies for Growing your Emotional Health.

1. Engage in physical activity to improve mood and decrease anxiety. Any type of exercise that you enjoy will get the endorphins flowing and help you feel better. This feel-good hormone is excellent for lifting spirits and helping people deal with depression.

2. Increase your circle of friends, you need people you can talk to about your problems. This will help you get things off your mind and remind you that you have people to back you up.

3. Educate yourself on whatever you're facing. This will help decrease the fear of the unknown. The more you know, the less you will fear what could happen.

4. Develop a new hobby. Humans are occupational beings, engaging in occupations relaxes your mind, gives you a sense of accomplishment, and helps boost your self-esteem.

5. Intimacy within a committed relationship has many psychological benefits. Having sex helps make you feel good about yourself and boosts your self-esteem.

6. Engage in activities for stress management including; meditation, yoga, or tai chi.

7. Eat healthy food, maintaining a healthy weight is important for your physical and emotional health.

8. Practice good time management by setting weekly goals. As you get things done, you'll feel a sense of accomplishment that will help relax you.

9. Take control of your life and make your own decisions.

10. Stay well-rested, when you are tired, everything can seem exaggerated, and even small problems will feel like big ones.

Chapter 26: How to Maintain Bone and Joint Health After an Injury

After healing from bone injuries it is common that you will have joint problems either in the short or long term. Your diet, genetics, or lifestyle may also cause different types of arthritis. Here are some tips for dealing with some of the most common joint disorders.

Detox

Although your body is built to detoxify itself, it was not configured to deal with industrial chemicals. The center for disease control (CDC) says that the typical person has, on average, 148 human-made toxic substances in their blood. Therefore, it is crucial to institute strategies on your own to help remove them from your body.

After surgery, your body could have a toxic accumulation of anesthesia, prescription medications, and other toxins. As part of your healing process, it's time to start taking time to remove blockages from your body caused by these toxins.

1. Eat organic fruits and vegetables and grass-fed animal proteins. Otherwise, you're taking in toxins at the same time that you're eliminating them, and never getting ahead.

2. Use natural body-care products, so you're not introducing new synthetic chemicals into your system. Keep toxins off your body; otherwise, it's the same as eating them.

3. Drink 3-4 glasses of water with freshly squeezed lemon first thing in the morning. Drinking water first thing in the morning will help clean out your bowels and flush out your liver. The more clean, filtered water you drink, the more you urinate, and the faster toxins leave your body.

4. Avoid cleaning products that contain carcinogens, reproductive system toxins, neurotoxins, and allergens. Use natural cleaning products to avoid all of these.

5. Avoid breathing in volatile organic compounds (VOC). Exposure to VOC's comes from paints, lacquers, thinners, glues, cleaning supplies, nail polish, markers, fuel, office equipment, inks, and pesticides. VOC's are up to ten times higher indoors than outdoors and can have short- and long-term health concerns.

6. Avoid using plastics as much as possible. Bisphenol A (BPA) is a hormone disruptor and has been found to cause disease in humans, including obesity and diabetes. Don't microwave plastics, use glass, or steel when possible instead, don't use plastic wraps and don't expose plastics to heat.

7. Use a sauna three times a week, up to twenty minutes at a time to sweat out toxins from your liver and fat tissue, to loosen joints, increase circulation, and reduce stiffness.

8. Supplement with minerals, which are critical for optimizing the detox pathways in the body. Two easy mineral-boosting strategies include; taking Epsom salt baths (for the magnesium) and drinking mineral water. Toxins such as heroin, cocaine, mercury, dioxin, and antibiotics can be removed from your body through sweat glands.

9. Eat the rainbow. The health-promoting compounds in vegetables and fruits are also usually responsible for their bright colors. The more colors you eat in a day, the more phytonutrients you'll get into your body. Phytonutrients assist with the detox process and help protect the body against more toxin-related damage. Try to eat one food from each color of the rainbow every day (red, orange, yellow, green, blue, purple). Enzymes from fruits and vegetables break down toxins in the liver.

10. Include some of the previously mentioned to help detox your system. Herbs such as ginger, dandelion, garlic, and parsley help optimize liver and kidney function.

11. Eat foods high in fiber to help toxins leave the body such as beans, oatmeal, avocados, berries, peas, squash, flax, and chia seeds.

12. Sleep is regenerative and can optimize all your body's functions, including its ability to detox.

13. Avoid genetically modified foods (GMO). Seventy to eighty percent of processed foods have GMO ingredients, while produce does not contain GMOs.

14. One to three-day juice cleanse allows your body to get the nutrients and caloric energy it needs, while allowing your digestive tract to rest, ingest max nutrients, minimize sugar and pollutant intake.

15. Gut bacteria is essential to overall health. Good bacteria are responsible for preventing many toxins from entering the body in the first place. Probiotic drinks like kefir, help provide healthy bacteria.

Chemicals to avoid in cosmetics and plastics. Many have been banned in Europe and in some U.S. states.

Toxin	Could be found in	Health Risk
Bisphenol A (BPA)	Resins, cosmetics, and plastics used in food and beverage containers.	Hormone disruptor, carcinogen
Pthalates	Plastics and nail polish	Hormone disruptor, carcinogen
Hydroquinone	Moisturizer, skin lightener	Hormone disruptor, carcinogen
Triclosan	Antibacterial soap	Hormone disruptor, carcinogen
Mercury	Eyedrops, skin	Neurotoxin,

	lightener	Hormone disruptor,
Coal Tar FD&C Blue 1 and Green 3	Mouthwash, toothpaste, dandruff shampoo, anti-itch cream	Carcinogen
Lead	Hair dye, lipstick	Hormone disruptor, carcinogen, neurotoxin
Diethanolamine (DEA)	Skin moisturizer, bath products	Hormone disruptor, carcinogen
P-Phenylenediami ne	Plastics, hair dye, foot powder	Hormone disruptor, carcinogen, allergen, neurotoxin
Butylated compounds (bht, bha)	Processed foods and cosmetics	Hormone disruptor, carcinogen,
Parabens	Processed foods and drugs	Hormone disruptor, carcinogen,
I, 4 Dioxane (PEG)	Laundry detergents, toothpaste, mouthwash, deodorant, bath products, and hair dyes.	Hormone disruptor, carcinogen,
Artificial	Variety of	Hormone

fragrance	consumer products	disruptor, carcinogen,
Quarternium-15 (Formaldehyde)	Nail polish, hair dye, bath gel	Hormone disruptor, carcinogen,
Toluene	Nail polish	Hormone disruptor, carcinogen, neurotoxin
Octinoxate	Cosmetics	Hormone disruptor
Siloxanes	Cosmetics	Hormone disruptor

Supplements for Liver Detox	Benefits
Minerals (Copper, zinc, selenium)	Helps the body make its own antioxidants and increases the efficiency of body functions.
B Vitamins	Supports improved liver and nervous system function.
Antioxidants (A, C, E)	Helps reduce the damage caused to your body from exposure to toxins.
SAMe (S-Adensyl-Methionine)	Helps with detoxifying the liver, decreases joint inflammation, and symptoms of depression.
NAC (N-acetyl-cysteine)	Helps with heavy metal

	exposure and respiratory disorders.
Milk Thistle	Protects and detoxes the liver.
Glycine	Helps with liver detox and reduces the damage to your liver caused by alcohol.
MSM (Methyl-sulf-Mathane)	Helps with liver function, joint problems, and decreases joint inflammation.
Lipoic acid	Helps increase circulation, especially in the liver
Supplements for Healthy Intestines	**Benefits**
Probiotics (Bifidophilus, acidophilus)	Helps improve digestion, intestinal function, and immune function.
Prebiotics (Beta-Glucan, Fructo-Oligo-Saccharides, Inulin)	Helps support growth of good bacteria and helps prevent bad ones.
L-glutamine	Helps repair the intestinal lining and improves nervous system function.
NAC/glutathione	Helps remove heavy metals from the body.

Product to avoid at home	**Toxic Chemicals**	**Health Risks**	**Alternative**

Kitchenware	PVC (plastic), Teflon	Hormone disruptor, carcinogen	Cast-iron pots and pans or steel. Glass storage containers instead of plastic
Mattress	PDBE (flame retardant), toluene, formaldehyde, polyurethane	Hormone disruptor, carcinogen, neurotoxin	Mattress encasement, natural cotton or wool filler, untreated mattress topper
Vinyl shower curtains	Release toxic plasticizer gases for up to 5 years	Hormone disruptor, carcinogen, neurotoxin	Cotton curtains
Carpet	Releases gases from adhesives, fire retardant, and stain proofing	Hormone disruptor, carcinogen, neurotoxin	Use VOC-free adhesives and natural carpet fibers; wool, jute, hemp, or sea grass
Cleaning products	TEA, DEA, bleach, chlorine, ammonia, acids, fragrances	Hormone disruptor, carcinogen, neurotoxin	Vinegar, borax, lemon juice, soap, water, baking soda,
Paints	Xylene, benzene,	Hormone disruptor,	Ventilate area, look

	formaldehyd e, toluene	carcinogen, neurotoxin	for no-VOC or low-VOC paint

Acupressure

Acupressure can increase blood flow to the muscles around the fracture or damaged joint, which can help the fracture heal faster or decrease discomfort in joint conditions. Here are some specific acupressure points to treat them.

A simple way to stimulate these points is to press firmly with a finger in a rotary movement or an up-and-down movement for several minutes at a time. Use this information under the guidance of your physician. Use deep, firm pressure to massage and stimulate each point.

1. LI11- Large intestine- LI11 located on the outer exterior side of the elbow which is the exterior area of the arm. Stimulating this point can treat simple fractures, provides relief from fever, joint discomfort, and skin diseases. Stimulate this point by applying mild pressure by you or someone else.

2. TW14 (Triple Warmer 14) – This acupressure point is located on the shoulder, posterior to LI 15, in a depression inferior and posterior to the acromion when arm is abducted. Stimulate this point by applying mild pressure by you or someone else.

3. LU9 (Lungs 9- LU9 located at the thin crease of the wrist. It is in line with the thumb and is good for repairing fractures near the arm. Hold the point with gentle pressure for 2 to 3 minutes.

4. TW15 (Triple Warmer 15)-The Triple Warmer Meridian originates from the tip of the ring finger, by the outside corner of the nail, passes between the knuckles of the fourth and fifth fingers, on to the wrist. From there it ascends between the two bones of the forearm (radius and ulna), through the tip of the elbow, and up the back of the arm to the shoulder, midway between the base of the neck and the outside of the shoulder, one-half inch below the top of the shoulder. If you gently apply pressure on this point with your thumb every day, then you can feel the pain disappears from fractured bones and joint discomfort. It also relieves nervous tension and stiff necks, increases resistance to colds and flu, and is good for the lungs.

5. SP6- This point is located 3 inches above the tip of the medial malleolus on the posterior border of the medial aspect of the tibia. Gently push this pressure point for a few minutes daily.

6. Sp7-This point is located 3 inches above SP5, on the line joining the tip of the medial malleolus and SP 9. Apply mild pressure on this point with your thumb for a few minutes, 3 to 4 times daily.

7. SP9– This point is located on the lower border of the medial condyle of tibia, in the depression in the medial border of the tibia.

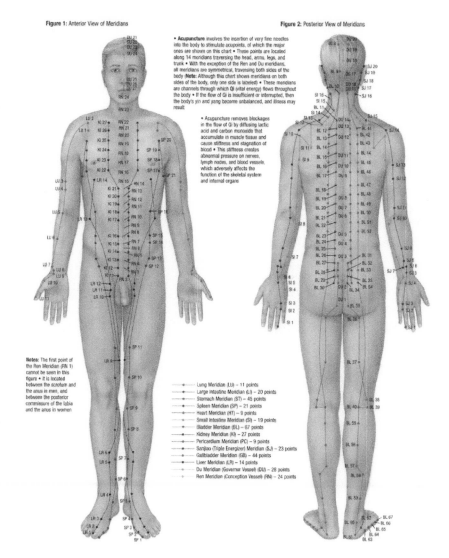

Figure 1: Anterior View of Meridians

Figure 2: Posterior View of Meridians

Acupuncture

Acupuncture is the insertion of very thin needles through your skin at natural energy points where the body's "Qi" can be stimulated. A key component of traditional Chinese medicine, acupuncture is most commonly used to treat pain and overall wellness. Acupuncture affects the autonomic nervous system (which controls bodily functions) and the release of chemicals that regulate blood flow and pressure, reduce inflammation, and has a calming effect on the brain.

Aromatherapy

Aromatic essential oils are extracted from plants, distilled, and mixed with other substances such as alcohol or lotion. They are then applied to the skin for absorption or sprayed into the air for inhaling. Inhaling a scent triggers powerful neurotransmitters and other chemicals that stimulate certain parts of the limbic system, which control emotions and behavior, resulting in an improved mood. Aromatherapy, also known as essential oil therapy, can enhance both physical and emotional health. Some of the benefits offered by aromatherapy include:

- pain management
- improved sleep quality
- reduce stress, agitation, and anxiety
- soothe sore joints
- treat headaches and migraines
- alleviate side effects of chemotherapy
- ease discomforts of labor
- fight bacteria, virus, or fungus
- improve digestion
- improve hospice and palliative care
- boost immunity.

Ayurveda

Ayurveda, also known as ayurvedic medicine means "knowledge of life," It's based on the belief that health and wellness depend on keeping the body and mind balanced and healthy.

Biofeedback

Biofeedback is a mind-body technique that involves using visual or auditory feedback to gain control over involuntary bodily functions. It includes gaining voluntary control over your heart rate, blood flow, muscle tension, pain perception, and blood pressure. By gaining control over some of these involuntary body functions you can speed up your healing and control symptoms such as pain.

Types of Biofeedback

1. Breathing: Respiratory biofeedback involves wearing sensor bands around the chest and abdomen to monitor breathing rates and patterns. With training, people can learn to have greater control over their breathing rates which can help in a variety of situations.

2. Heart rate: This type is known as heart rate variability biofeedback and there is some evidence that it might possibly be useful for a number of different disorders including asthma and depression. Patients using this type of biofeedback wear a device connected to sensors in either the ears or fingers or sensors placed on the wrists, chest, or torso. These devices measure heart rate as well as heart rate variability.

3. Galvanic skin response: This type of biofeedback involves measuring the amount of sweat on the surface of the skin. Galvanic skin response, also known as skin conductance, is a useful marker for detecting levels of emotional arousal. Aside from the obvious thermoregulatory function of sweat, emotional stimulation can also easily trigger sweating. The more strongly people are aroused, the stronger their skin conductance will be.

4. Blood pressure: This type of biofeedback involves wearing a device that measures blood pressure. These devices provide information about the patient's blood pressure and often guide the user through relaxation techniques that may rely on visual cues, breathing exercises, or music. While such devices have gained popularity, one study reviewing eight previous trials did not find convincing evidence that this type of biofeedback has any lasting long-term impact on hypertension.

5. Skin temperature: In this form of biofeedback, patients wear sensors that detect blood flow to the skin. Because people often experience a drop in body temperature during times of stress, such devices can help people better detect

169

when they are starting to feel distressed. A low reading on one of these monitors can indicate a need to utilize some stress management techniques.

6. Brain waves: This type of biofeedback, often referred to as neurofeedback, involves utilizing electroencephalography (EEG) to measure brain wave activity. Scalp sensors are connected to an EEG device. Neurofeedback is sometimes used as a non-invasive treatment for ADHD, pain, addiction, anxiety, depression, and other disorders.

7. Muscle tension: In this type of biofeedback, sensors are placed at various points on the body and connected to an electromyography (EMG) device. This device detects changes in muscle tension over time by monitoring electrical activity that results in muscle contractions.

CBD Oil

Cannabidiol (CBD) oil is a naturally found chemical in marijuana plants. CBD oil is extracted from the cannabis plant, then diluted with a carrier oil like hemp seed or coconut oil. CBD oil does not contain tetrahydrocannabinol (THC) which is the primary psychoactive cannabinoid found in cannabis, and causes the feeling of getting "high" that comes from marijuana. However, CBD is not psychoactive, like THC, which makes CBD appealing for people who are looking for relief from pain and other symptoms without the mind-altering effects of marijuana or other pharmaceutical drugs. CBD has helped people avoid using medications like benzodiazepines which can be addictive and can lead to substance abuse. I've seen dozens of patients, and medical colleagues that have treated joint problems with CBD oil and many patients report being able to avoid pain medications altogether after surgeries by using CBD oil.

CBD oil has been used to treat chronic pain, anxiety, depression, inflammation, insomnia, post-traumatic stress disorder, lower blood pressure, acne, neurological disorders like epilepsy and multiple sclerosis, regulate mood and social behavior, and diabetes. CBD can help reduce symptoms related to cancer and side effects related to cancer treatment, like nausea, vomiting, and pain. CBD can also be used to treat different forms of cancer. In drug rehabilitation, CBD is used to reduce addictive behaviors and reduce psychotic symptoms in psychiatric patients.

Clinical research has shown CBD to help heal bone fractures, speed up the process and make bones stronger.

CBD oil is generally safe and has few side effects including; diarrhea, changes in appetite and weight, and fatigue.

Check your state's laws and those of anywhere you travel before carrying CBD oil across state lines. Marijuana-derived CBD products are illegal on the federal level but are legal in some states. Hemp-derived CBD products (with less than 0.3 percent THC) are permitted on the national level but are still illegal under some state laws.

Flotation Tank

The Flotation tank, also known as a sensory deprivation tank, is filled with water that is heated to skin temperature and saturated with Epsom salt (magnesium sulfate), providing buoyancy so you float more easily. You enter the tank naked then close the tank's lid and are cut off from all outside stimulation, including sound, sight, and gravity.

While floating in the tank, your body absorbs the magnesium sulfate, which helps calm your nervous system and enhances your body's natural ability to heal. Your cortisol levels are also lowered as you enter a deep state of relaxation.

Flower Essence

In the 1930s, Dr. Edward Bach created the flower essence system. Flower therapy, or essence therapy, is considered vibrational medicine, based on the idea that everything in nature, including flowers and your own body, has its own vibration. When vibration is out of tune in the body, which can be caused by emotional distress and illness, using flower essences with its specific vibration can help restore calm and balance.

Distilled essences of wildflowers, which are liquids infused with a flower's energy, are usually preserved in an alcohol base and administered internally, under the tongue, to balance your emotions. The goal in vibrational medicine is to move, unblock or balance life energy over the physical, energetic, and spiritual body. Doing so will help bring about mental, physical, and spiritual wellness.

Flower essences are water-based, made only from flowers. On the other hand, aromatherapy essential oils are oil-based and made from the aromatic parts of plants. The main difference is flower essences are typically taken internally with an eyedropper. You can add them to your water bottle and sip throughout the day. In contrast, essential oils are applied topically or inhaled.

Food Therapy

Using specific foods to heal specific ailments. For example, eating bone broth and extra protein to help heal a fractured bone.

Herbal Therapy

Herbal medicine uses medicinal plants for herbal therapy. Plants are used for medical treatments.

Homeopathy

Homeopathy uses homeopathic medicines made from plants, chemical, mineral or animal sources. These medicines are used to treat physical and psychological ailments.

Massage

Massage therapy is the manual manipulation of soft body tissues (muscle, connective tissue, tendons, and ligaments) to enhance a person's health and well-being. Massage techniques are commonly applied with hands, feet, fingers, forearms, elbows, knees, or a device. The purpose of massage is generally for treating body stress, pain, or increasing circulation.

Nutrition Therapy

Nutrition therapy is a medical approach to treating medical conditions using tailored diet plans devised and monitored by a medical doctor physician or registered dietitian nutritionist.

Physiatrists

Physical Medicine and Rehabilitation (PM&R) doctors, also known as physiatrists, treat a wide variety of medical conditions affecting the brain, spinal cord, nerves, bones, joints, ligaments, muscles, and tendons.

Poultice

A poultice is a soft moist mass, often heated and medicated, that is spread on cloth over the skin to treat an inflamed, aching, or painful part of the body.

Relaxation Therapy

Relaxation therapy helps reduce muscle tension and stress, control pain, and lower blood pressure. A relaxation technique is any method, procedure, process, or activity that helps a person to relax, increase calmness, or reduce levels of pain, anxiety, anger, or stress.

Thermal Biofeedback

Thermal biofeedback, also known as psychophysiological feedback, uses a person's body temperature to assess that person's physical state. Thermal biofeedback works by attaching a temperature sensor or thermistor to a patient, normally the hands or fingers. A digital screen shows a temperature readout of the patient, who can track their body temperature by the minute.

Reflexology

Reflexology is a type of massage that involves applying different amounts of pressure to the feet, hands, or ears. Reflexologists believe that applying pressure to these body parts offers health benefits because they're connected to certain organs and body systems.

Biomagnetism

Biomagnetism is a magnetic field produced by living organisms. Biomagnetism treatment involves the precise and proper (North/South polarity) placement of special high field strength magnets over specific areas of the body, to cause regulation of pH levels in those areas. By balancing pH levels, homeostasis can be reestablished so the body can heal itself.

This treatment stimulates normal immune system function, increases circulation, oxygenation, and normalizes response to inflammation. Imbalances in pH can accumulate and cause the development of symptoms, syndromes and other health conditions in our bodies. By reestablishing the natural pH balance of the body, microorganisms such as viruses, fungi, bacteria, and parasites can be kept under control by our renewed natural defenses.

Alexander Technique

The Alexander technique teaches you how to improve your posture and movement, which helps reduce and prevent problems caused by bad habits. Treatment focuses on teaching you to be more aware of your body, how to improve poor posture, and increase the efficiency of movement.

Feldenkrais Method

The Feldenkrais Method works with your nervous system to make changes in your movements. By retraining your brain, your nervous system will change the way it directs your body to move more efficiently.

Progressive Relaxation

Progressive Muscle Relaxation (PMR) used to reduce body tension and psychological stress. By repeatedly tensing your muscles and then relaxing them, your muscles will progressively relax more and more after each release. This process helps release physical tension and relax your body

Hydrotherapy; Hot/Cold Contrast Bath

Hydrotherapy is also known as aquatic therapy, water therapy, pool therapy, and balneotherapy. Water is used externally or internally in different forms (water, ice, steam) to promote or treat various diseases with various temperatures, pressure, duration, and site. Hydrotherapy improves many health disorders, including; immunity, manages pain, cardiac problems, respiratory issues, circulatory disorders, fatigue, anxiety, obesity, hypercholesterolemia, labor, and hyperthermia. The results vary depending on the temperature of the water and how it is applied.

Hot/Cold contrast baths are a therapeutic treatment where a portion of the entire body is immersed first in hot water, then in ice water. By alternating immersion into hot and cold several times. You can improve circulation around injured tissue.

Myofascial Release

Myofascial Release is a manual therapy technique that uses sustained pressure into the myofascial connective tissue to reduce or eliminate restrictions in movement. By doing so you can improve skeletal muscle mobility, stimulate the stretch reflex in muscles, reduce pain by relaxing contracted muscles, and improve blood and lymphatic circulation.

Shaolin Medicine

Shaolin Chan Medicine can be traced to the Shaolin Temple in China. It is a monastery where monks practice martial arts, meditate, and practice Shaolin. The philosophy of Shaolin includes energy, healing, physical conditioning, control, balance, flexibility, speed, agility, and power. Over time the monks began to accumulate medical experience by taking advantage of abundant herbal resources in the Song Mountain and benefitting from the folk medical approaches. They developed Qigong therapy, massage therapy and pointing therapy which is used for medical treatments. Shaolin Medicine can treat various diseases, treat traumatic injuries, and has many divisions such as surgery and internal departments.

Applied Kinesiology

Applied Kinesiology (AK) is a non-invasive system of evaluating body functions, as well as chemical, structural, and mental aspects of health using manual muscle testing to evaluate body function through the dynamics of the musculoskeletal systems in combination with other standard methods of diagnosis. Treatments can involve joint manipulation or mobilization, clinical nutrition, dietary management, myofascial therapies, cranial techniques, various reflex procedures, meridian and acupuncture skills, counseling skills, and evaluating environmental irritants.

Occupational and Physical Therapy

Physical therapists, also known as PTs, treat injured, disabled, or sick people to improve their movement and manage their pain. Therapists are an important part of rehabilitation, treatment, and prevention of patients with chronic conditions, illnesses, or injuries.

Occupational therapists, also known as OTs, treat injured, disabled, or sick people through the therapeutic use of everyday activities.

Osteoarthritis

Osteoarthritis, also known as OA, is the most common form of arthritis, affecting millions of people worldwide (over 3 million new cases a year in the U.S.). It occurs when the protective cartilage that cushions the ends of your bones wears down and worsens over time. Joint pain and loss of mobility are the main symptoms. OA can damage any joint, but it most commonly affects joints in your hands, knees, hips, and spine. If you've ever fractured, sprained, dislocated, or had any other type of trauma to a bone or joint, there is an increased risk of developing OA in the future in that area.

Osteoarthritis symptoms can usually be managed, but the damage to joints can't be reversed. Ways to manage OA include: staying active and maintaining a healthy body weight. The treatments outlined below will slow the progression of the disease and help decrease pain and improve joint function.

OA symptoms develop slowly and worsen over time. Signs and symptoms of osteoarthritis include:

- Burning pain in affected joints which exacerbates during or after movement.

- Joint stiffness, which is usually more noticeable after being inactive i.e. After you wake up in the mornings

- A popping/crackling sound during movement

- The joint may feel tender when you apply light pressure to or near it.

- Loss of full range of motion and flexibility.

- A grating sensation when using the joint

- Formation of extra bits of bone around the affected joint. These hard lumps are called bone spurs and can cause more discomfort during movement as they grind into your body tissue.

- Soft tissue inflammation can cause swelling around the affected joint.

Treatment for Osteoarthritis

Traditional Treatment	**Alternative Treatment**

Acetaminophens	Acupressure; st 36 points
Topical analgesics; Capsaicin, Salicylates, menthol, methyl salicylate (oil of evergreen), and camphor,	Acupuncture Topical CBD Oil
Aspirin	Aromatherapy; rosemary or chamomile essentials
Nonsteroidal anti-inflammatory drugs (NSAIDS); Aspirin (Bufferin, Bayer), Celecoxib (Celebrex), Diclofenac (Cataflam, Voltaren), Diflunisal (Dolobid), Etodolac (Lodine), Fenoprofen (Nalfon) Flurbiprofen (Ansaid), Ibuprofen (Advil, Motrin)	SAM-e Ayurveda; sesame oil, spicy herbs
Heat Therapy; ultrasound, diathermy, hot pack, hot bath, hot tub	Biofeedback
Cold Treatments; ice packs	Flotation Tanks
Exercise; walking, swimming, stationary bike	Food Therapy; green veggies, low-fat diet
Corticosteroids; Corticosteroids; hydrocortisone (Cortef), cortisone, ethamethasoneb (Celestone), prednisone (Prednisone Intensol), prednisolone (Orapred, Prelone), triamcinolone	Herbal therapy; devil's claw tea, comfrey, valerian, black cohosh, chaparral, yucca, celery seed, boswellia serrata, pycogenol

(Aristospan Intra-Articular, Aristospan Intralesional, Kenalog) Methylprednisolone (Medrol, Depo-Medrol, Solu-Medrol)	
Occupational Therapy; energy conservation training, adaptive equipment	Homeopathy; rhus toxicodendron, arnica, cimicifuga
Surgery; joint replacement, arthroscopic procedures	Massage
	Nutritional therapy; dietary supplements
	Physiatry
	Poultice; Epsom salts
	Relaxation therapy; stretch therapy
	Thermal Biofeedback
	Shaolin Medicine

Treatments for Rheumatoid Arthritis

Rheumatoid arthritis (RA) is an autoimmune disease that causes the body's immune system to mistakenly attack its joints instead of simply doing its normal job of protecting the body's health by attacking foreign substances like bacteria and viruses. This process causes inflammation that causes the tissue that lines the inside of joints (the synovium) to thicken, resulting in swelling and pain in and around the joints. The synovium makes a fluid that lubricates joints and helps them move smoothly.

If the inflammation is not addressed it can damage cartilage and the bones themselves. Over time cartilage is eroded, the joint spacing between bones can become smaller, joints can become loose, unstable, painful, lose their mobility, and become deformed. Joint damage cannot be reversed, therefore it is important to treat it early and aggressively.

Traditional Treatment	Alternative Treatment
Aspirin	Acupressure
Nonsteroidal anti-inflammatory drugs (NSAIDS); aspirin salsalate (Amigesic), diflunisal (Dolobid), ibuprofen (Motrin), ketoprofen (Orudis), nabumetone (Relafen), piroxicam (Feldene), naproxen (Aleve, Naprosyn,) diclofenac (Voltaren), indomethacin (Indocin), sulindac (Clinoril), tolmetin (Tolectin), etodolac (Lodine), ketorolac (Toradol), oxaprozin (Daypro), celecoxib (Celebrex).	Acupuncture
Gastrointestinal Medications; Antacids, Aluminum hydroxide, magnesium hydroxide (Mylanta, Maalox), Calcium carbonate (Tums, Rolaids, Chooz), Proton Pump	Fish Oil

Inhibitors, Omeprazole (Prilosec), Lansoprazole (Prevacid), Histamine2 Blockers, Cimetidine (Tagamet), Ranitidine hydrochloride (Zantac), Promotility Agents, Metoclopramide (Reglan)	
Disease-Modifying antirheumatic drugs (DMARDS); methotrexate, sulfasalazine, hydroxychloroquine, and leflunomide. Less frequently used medications include gold salts, azathioprine, and cyclosporine.	Flotation Tank
Immunosuppressants; nitrogen mustard (1-3), azathioprine (4-9), 6-mercaptopurine (9-11), chlorambucil (12-14), cyclophosphamide (15), and methotrexate (16).	Food: vegetarian, reduced-fat diet
Corticosteroids: hydrocortisone (Cortef), cortisone, ethamethasoneb (Celestone), prednisone (Prednisone Intensol), prednisolone (Orapred, Prelone), triamcinolone (Aristospan Intra-Articular, Aristospan Intralesional, Kenalog) Methylprednisolone (Medrol, Depo-Medrol, Solu-Medrol)	Herbal Therapy: celery seed, wild yam, dandelion, lignum vitae.

Surgery: synovectomy, arthrodesis, tendon transfer, arthroplasty	Homeopathy, bryonia, cimicifuga, rhus toxicodendron
Exercise: range of motion, walking, swimming, stationary bike, endurance, aerobic, strengthening	Hydrotherapy, moist heat packs, cold wet compress, contrast bath
Occupational Therapy: energy conservation, joint protection, stress management, adaptive equipment, assistive equipment, splinting	Imagery
	Juice Therapy using: Parsely, broccoli, spinach, carrot, ginger, apple
	Massage, effleurage stroke
	Physiatry
	Nutritional Therapy including: vitamin E, Vitamin C, bromelain, selenium, zinc, copper, borage oil
	Yoga
	Shaolin Medicine

Treatments for Bursitis

Bursae are fluid-filled sacs that act as a cushion between bones, tendons, joints, and muscles. When these sacs become inflamed it is called bursitis. Bursitis causes severe joint pain during functional tasks. Tennis elbow is a type of bursitis.

Traditional Treatment	Alternative Treatment
RICE; rest, ice, compression, and elevation	Acupuncture
Nonsteroidal anti-inflammatory drugs (NSAIDS); aspirin, ibuprofen (Advil, Nuprin).	Castor oil Treatment
Corticosteroids; local anesthetic	Food therapy; pineapple, barley greens
Fluid withdrawal	Homeopathy; calcarea flourica, bryonia, benzoic acid, rhus toxicodendron, ruta grav.
Surgery	Herbal tea; chamomile, passion flower, skullcap, lady's slipper
Heat Treatments; heating pad, warm moist cloth	Massage Therapy
Ultrasound therapy	Nutritional therapy; calcium, magnesium, vitamins A, C, E
Exercise	Poultices
	Reflexology
	Shaolin Medicine

Treatment for Gout

Gout is a type of arthritis caused by excessive uric acid in the bloodstream. Over time uric acid crystals start to form in the joints and it causes pain, redness, swelling, and inflammation. The big toe is the most commonly affected joint in the body. The best treatment for gout is behavioral modification such as diet, exercise, and decreased intake of alcohol to help minimize the frequency of attacks. Every person will have specific diet related triggers for their gout. Pay attention to what foods, preservatives, or seasonings cause your flare ups and exclude those particular items from your diet.

Traditional Treatment	Alternative Treatment
Medication; Allopurinol (Aloprim, Zyloprim) reduces uric acid production, Colchicine (Colcrys) reduces inflammation, Febuxostat (Uloric) reduces uric acid production, Indomethacin (Indocin) is a stronger NSAID pain reliever.	Acupuncture; spleen, liver, large intestine
Bed Rest; elevated bedding	Aromatherapy; juniper/rosemary footbath
Lifestyle Changes; Limit alcohol consumption, reduce stress, lose excessive weight	Nutritional Therapy; limit fats, sugars, avoid meats, gravies, sugar, white flour, cakes, pies, beans, fish, cauliflower, lentils, oatmeal, peas, poultry, yeast, and spinach
	Herbal teas; peppermint, yarrow, sarsaparilla
	Herbal therapy; willow bark, celery seed, silver

	birch
	Homeopathy; aconite, urtica urens, colchicum, belladonna, ledum 30, nux vomica
	Hydrotherapy; cold compress, ice pack, charcoal foot soak
	Reflexology; kidney point #25
	Biofeedback; blood pressure reduction
	Juice therapy; tart cherry
	Nutritional Therapy; Vitamin A and C, Niacin restrictions
	Shaolin Medicine

Treatment for Sprains

A sprain is the tearing of ligaments in a joint, often caused by trauma or the joint being taken beyond its functional range of motion. The more tearing that occurs the more profound the sprain will be.

Traditional Treatments	Alternative Treatments
RICE; Rest, ice, compression, elevation	Comfrey poultice, compress
Heat	Herbal therapy; Arnica, burdock, ginger tea

Pain relievers; analgesics, aspirin	Acupressure
surgery	Food Therapy; grapefruit, oranges, strawberries, peppers
	Ayurveda; salt, turmeric
	Homeopathy; arnica, ruta graveolens, rhus toxicodendron
	Massage; rake technique
	Herbal supplements; bromelain, curcumin
	Nutritional Therapy; vitamin C, magnesium, proteolytic enzymes, amino acids, B12, B6
	Reflexology
	Electrotherapy
	Ultrasound
	Yoga
	Menthol
	Folk remedies; oil of wintergreen, tofu, orange peel, vinegar, onions
	Shaolin Medicine
	Applied Kinesiology

Treatment for Dislocations

A dislocation is an injury to a joint where two adjoining bones are forced from their normal condition. This type of injury is painful and temporarily deforms and immobilizes the joint. Dislocation happens most commonly in the shoulders and fingers.

Traditional Treatments	Alternative Treatments
Emergency medical care	Homeopathy; symphytum, rescue remedy, arnica
Physical and Occupational Therapy	Herbal treatment; salves or ointments, comfrey poultice or compress
	Biomagnetism

Treatment for Bunion

A bunion, also known as hallux valgus, is a bony deformity of the joint at the base of the big toe. As the toe becomes deformed, a bony, swollen, painful, bump forms on the outside edge of your foot. The pain increases whenever pressure from wearing shoes is applied.

Traditional Treatment	Alternative Treatment
Footwear	Acupressure; Lv3 point
Orthotics; mass-produced, custom fit	Arch support
Surgery; open technique, closed technique	Aromatherapy; juniper, lavender oils

	Aspirin Wrap
	Barefoot walking
	Food therapy
	Heating Pad
	Homeopathy; strontium carbonicum, zeel, apis, sulphur, ruta graveolens
	Lotions and bath oils
	Massage
	Stretched shoes
	Nutrition Therapy
	Pads, separation, moleskin, or sling pad
	Shaolin Medicine

Treatment for Carpal Tunnel Syndrome

Carpal tunnel syndrome occurs when nerves in the wrist, mainly the median nerve is compressed as it travels through the wrist. It is becoming more common as people work more and more on computers. Common symptoms include; pain, numbness, and tingling in the hand and arm.

Traditional Treatment	Alternative treatment
Rest	Acupuncture
Splints	Nutrition Therapy; B, C, E

Medications	Acupressure
	Alexander technique
	Feldenkrais Method
	Homeopathy; cimicifuga, rhus toxicodendron, bryonia
	Progressive relaxation
	Hydrotherapy; hot/cold contrast bath
	Myofascial release
	Shaolin Medicine
	Applied Kinesiology

Chapter 27: How to Financially Survive a Broken Bone

Surviving a trauma is going to be one of the most impactful events in your life. The choices you make will have lifelong repercussions. In most cases not only is there physical suffering ahead but financial. With good care and dedication to a treatment plan as outlined in this book you'll be able to recover from the physical aspects of the injury, but the financial damage can often times put all aspects of your life into a downward tailspin.

In my case, and for many of the patients I treat, even as you lay in a hospital bed wondering if you're going to survive, you're inevitably going to start thinking about your finances and what lies ahead. It seems as if it would be the last thing that you would be thinking about when you're facing possible death, in lots of pain, and in fear of the possible outcomes, but in reality, it's a very practical matter to be concerned about, as often times you've already worked your entire life to build up your career, your finances, and accumulated possessions that have made your life more comfortable. One injury can easily take all of that away and wipe out your life's work.

Luckily when I had my injury, I had an idea of the financial stress coming my way mostly from the numerous patients that I have met and treated over twenty years of practice. Each had explained to me in detail how their financial empire was crumbling before their very eyes and there was nothing they could do because they were bed-bound due to an illness or injury.

In my case, my orthopedic surgeon was prescribing six months of bed rest with no-weight bearing and two years of being in a wheelchair after that. This was my best case scenario based on whether or not I would survive the operations or the recovery process. I have a family that I help support financially, who would also be put into a financial disaster if I wasn't able to continue assisting financially. Your injury can also jeopardize the people who depend on you.

Thankfully, I had some idea of what needed to be done to survive, and the rest I learned as the process of recovery unfolded. In general, I believe it's best to keep your financial house in order all the time. In fact, one of the reasons you want to do so, is to survive all the uncertainty that comes your way when an unexpected event occurs.

Insurance

Insurance is going to be your first line of defense and probably the most vital. Without insurance you will absorb more risk than is necessary. Risk is a part of life; however, insurance gives you a way to lower that risk. Let's use an analogue to explain why we need insurance. Think about fastening your seatbelt after getting in the car. Wearing a seatbelt doesn't mean you'll get in an accident nor does it mean that you'll survive an accident. However, wearing a seatbelt does increase the probability that you'll survive an accident and it does decrease the risk of sustaining an injury. Therefore, it is good practice to wear a seatbelt when you get into a car. Insurance works the same way and it can help prevent almost certain financial ruin for over 90% of people. Below are some of the most commonly available types of insurance listed by importance.

Shop around to get the best rates on the different types of insurance. Usually the more you pay the more coverage you'll get, but if you're financially strapped, get at least the minimum so you have some coverage in case of an unexpected accident, and so you can get preventative medical care. Often times if people would simply get yearly physicals and blood tests, they could avoid having more severe medical problems in the future by maintaining their current health.

Health Insurance

Having health insurance is the foundation for any financial or life plan for several reasons. First, the cost of healthcare is astronomical, I personally accumulated over

$200,000 in debt after being in the hospital for 12 days, and that was just the beginning of my care. I ended up needing treatments and medical care for almost two years after my injury. If I would have not had health insurance I would have owed all of that money, my credit would have been ruined, the hospitals would sue me for the money, my assets could have been seized by a court to settle the debts, liens could have been placed on my assets, wages could have been garnished, family could have been left destitute, and all of my life's savings would have been used to pay the debts. I've personally met patients who have explained to me in detail how they were once wealthy, lost everything due to illness or injury, and either live in the streets or live completely dependent on government support. Just as an example, a spinal cord injury can cost over two million dollars in the first year of care and several million after that to keep you alive.

Secondly, uninsured people receive less medical care and less timely care, and have worse health outcomes. When I was studying and training at a county hospital in Los Angeles, we were told that the first thing the patient or accompanying family member had to do when they arrived was to sign in because the hospital needs the patient to agree to their clauses before they would start treatment. One of the most important clauses in the agreement was that the hospital had 72 hours before they may start giving you medical care. This protects them from being sued in case you come in and you happen to die while waiting to be seen. This seemed harsh at first, but after I started seeing the ocean of uninsured people coming in, I started to understand. I had seen some of the worst accidents I've ever seen in my life. Many had gunshot wounds or had been stabbed. In fact, during the Iraq and Afghanistan wars, the U.S. military would send their doctors to the county hospital in Los Angeles to prepare them for the battlefields. As a result of the large unexpected influxes of patients, hospitals use a triage system similar to what is used on the battlefield. They basically see the patients that have the highest probability of surviving first and invest less time and resources into treating patients that are less likely to survive or are uninsured. Therefore, a person who could have possibly made a full recovery from a stroke may end up with paraplegia or other lingering deficits from their stroke as a result of being treated several hours or days after they initially reported to the hospital. After being treated and stabilized if you don't have insurance the hospital will release you and you're on your own to figure out how to rehabilitate yourself from whatever injury or illness you have. This leaves thousands of people with lifelong disabilities and unable to physically work to support themselves. Unfortunately, this is something that many people don't understand. You can not go back and treat or rehabilitate an injury after time passes as the damage has become permanent. For example, after you are stabilized from suffering a stroke, you have an approximate window of about 6-12 months where the treatments you receive can have a big outcome on your recovery. Day by day that window closes so the therapy you receive three months after the injury is not as impactful as the treatment you could have received one month after and so on. When it comes to bones, if you don't treat the injury properly the bone will heal in whatever position it's in, so going back to fix the damage a couple of months later might require rebreaking the bone and trying to help it heal properly. This would cause you to have to relive the trauma twice and cause you to miss work twice as long.

Consider the alternative, where you are insured and instead of going to the overcrowded county hospitals you can go to a private hospital where the staff would possibly have more time to treat you and they won't be burdened with having to just stabilize you and kick you out the door. Instead, they could make a proper treatment plan that includes consults from various medical specialists as needed, access to the best medical facilities, aftercare, rehabilitation services, and even home care as needed to make sure you reach your optimal function after your injury. In my case my physicians told my leg would have been amputated if I would have gone to a county hospital and/or have been uninsured.

If you want to be successful in life, build wealth, or even

193

just live a long healthy life, do not try to save money by passing up health insurance if you can afford it. The benefits of coverage, far outweigh the costs.

If you are injured, you'll have fewer options available, but you'll still have some.

You can try negotiating the debt with the hospital, hospitals can sometimes forgive all of the debt if you can prove that you have no assets. They can reduce the amount you owe and offer you payment plans. In many cases some of the doctors you'll be seeing are not in your insurance network, therefore their treatments are not covered by your insurance which leaves you having to pay the doctor's bill even when you have health insurance. In my case my surgeons were covered but my anesthesiologists were not. Therefore, every time I had a surgery the anesthesiologists charged me $1500. Since I had four surgeries, I ended up owing $6000 in medical bills. This is a loophole that saves the insurance companies money and makes the doctors more. If you have the time, request doctors in your network and if you end up with some that aren't in your network as I did, you can try negotiating down the bill.

Some states also have financial assistance available to people who are a victim of a crime. In these cases, the state may step in and pick up the cost of your medical care. If other parties are involved, the other party may also have some type of insurance that will pay for your medical care. Remember most insurance policies whether its car insurance or some other type of insurance have liability coverage that can pay for your medical care. Cities often have free or subsidized community health clinics, and universities have discounted or free medical services available so that their students can practice.

After you have exhausted all of your options and you still need medical care, treating yourself may be an option if you have no others. YouTube has experts in everything you can think of, explaining step by step how to treat disorders. I personally did hundreds of hours of library and internet research reading about my broken leg and how best to treat it. Many of the strategies in this book are based on my research.

Another cost saving option is medical tourism. You can get the same medical care and even better in some cases for much less in other countries. I personally had two lipomas (fatty tumors) removed by a surgeon in Los Angeles who charged me over $20,000 for an outpatient procedure. I went to Mexico and had the others removed for $250 by a surgeon in Mexico. I've had other medical treatments for myself and family done abroad for the excellent savings they present and the quality of care. If you're considering medical tourism do your research and consider some of the best hospitals which often are rated higher than most US hospitals. Most international hospitals offer excellent medical care, require that all of their patient care staff speak English, and offer amenities like a luxury hotel.

Some of the world's best medical tourism hospitals;

1. Bumrungrad International, Thailand

2. Prince Court Medical Center, Malaysia

3. Asklepios Klinik Barmbek, Germany

4. Asian Heart Institute, India

5. Clemenceau Medical Center, Lebanon

6. Fortis Hospital Bangalore, India

7. Wooridul Spine Hospital, Korea

8. Gleneagles Hospital, Singapore

9. Anadolu Medical Center, Turkey

10. Bangkok Hospital Medical Center, Thailand

Disability Insurance

Private disability insurance will provide you a source of income if are unable to work due to an accident or illness.

Most people don't buy this type of insurance, but it's very useful in case you ever get hurt. Most plans cover 50-75% of your income in case of an injury. In most cases this can be more than your regular pay. Since disability payments are non-taxable, no taxes are subtracted from your payments, and you don't have to pay at the end of the year when you file your taxes. It's basically tax-free income. I've had patients who were on disability for years at a time and the insurance is usually very affordable.

Unions often offer discounted private disability insurance and are able to negotiate a price for all of their union members.

Some states (California, Hawaii, New Jersey, New York, Rhode Island, and the territory of Puerto Rico) offer state disability insurance (SDI), which subtracts around 1% of your yearly wages as a payroll deduction. If you ever get hurt or sick, you can apply for state disability benefits. As an example, in California weekly benefits range from $50 to a maximum of $1,252 for 52 weeks. In order for your state disability to be active you have to have worked at least one day in the last two years This will allow you to collect benefits for up to two years after working that job. The weekly amount you get paid will depend on your wages and generally lasts a maximum of 52 weeks. Benefits are also available to self-employed people as elective coverage and are paid for a maximum of 39 weeks.

Depending on the state, there are also other forms of financial aid available such as food stamps, general relief, housing assistance, permanent disability (federal), and free legal assistance for a person who is in jail. Some are asset-based, but others like the free legal assistance are for people who are on any type of government assistance including state disability.

Workers Compensation Insurance

Workers' compensation insurance, insures employees for illnesses and injuries that happen as a result of their job. Depending on state rules, injured employees receive a portion of their wages while they are off work for the treatment of their injury or illness.

As an example, in California you can receive up to 104 weeks of workers' comp benefits in a five-year period. That period starts the day of the injury. Some injuries such as severe burns and chronic lung disease qualify workers for 240 weeks of benefits. The injured worker is entitled to receive two-thirds of his pretax gross wages. The maximum rate in 2019 is $1,215.27 per week for a total disability, while the minimum paid is $182.29.

Unemployment Insurance

Unemployment insurance programs are set up by federal and state agencies to provide eligible employees with benefits when they lose their jobs. Employees must be out of work through no fault of their own, and meet certain eligibility requirements.

Student Loans

Contact your lenders and ask what options they have available. Some of the options available are;

1. Graduated Payment Plan. Some lenders will lower payments while you're recovering from your injury and increase them later on when you're back to work.

2. Income-Based Repayment Plan. Your loans can be adjusted based on the temporary drop in your income.

3. Deferment. If you have not defaulted on previous payments, you can defer your loan payments for a set period of time. Deferment is usually allowed if you go back to school, you're having difficulty making payments due to unemployment, or you're having other financial problems.

4. Forbearance. If you are unable to make payments due to your injury the lender may allow you to stop making payments for a specified period of time.

5. Extended Repayment Plan. You can also change the

terms of your loan. Standard student loan repayment plans allow for payment over the course of 10 years. Some lenders may allow you to change the terms of your loan repayment program so your payments are made over 25 years.

Home Mortgage Loans

If you're having trouble making your payments due to your injury, contact your loan servicer and ask about alternative repayment plans. Your servicer can give you reduced payments if you can't afford your mortgage payment because of financial hardship, like a job loss or medical bills.

The same type of options may be available with other lenders such as credit cards and personal loans if you have suffered a medical emergency.

Retirement Accounts

Most retirement accounts including 401k, 403b, and IRAs allow for hardship withdrawals if you've suffered a medical emergency. Many also allow you to borrow against the account for 60 days without any questions asked and no penalties.

Create a Budget and Financial Plan.

Creating and keeping a budget will allow you to balance your spending and saving, help ensure that you have enough money available for the things that are important to you, and to help you reach your goals. Budgets also help you stay out of debt, or help you get out of debt if you're in debt.

A financial plan tells you how to spend and invest the money you have budgeted to reach business goals. When driving somewhere that you're not familiar with, you use a map, or a mapping application, to get to your desired destination. This helps you get there the fastest, safest, and most efficient way possible. Without a financial plan, you're going to waste money, make it much slower than you probably could, and put your money at unnecessary risk.

Create a budget with your current income and liabilities. Then make a written financial plan with short and long term financial goals that you can reference regularly. Having a business plan will give you a map to reference and to help you stay on the right path. It's like using a workout routine when you go to the gym. Without a plan, you can get hurt from overtraining, or not get the physique you want for the beach.

One strategy to use is the 50-30-20 method. Senator Elizabeth Warren helped develop this plan while at Harvard. The biggest piece, 50% of your take-home income, should go towards essentials and basic living expenses; food, housing, and transportation. The second is 30% for flexible spending on discretionary expenses; clothing, travel, and entertainment. The last 20% goes towards helping you meet your financial goals of paying down debt and saving.

First, look at all your sources of income and determine how much you have available to spend each month. This will be your total income and this is what you're going to divide up into your 50/30/20 budget plan. If you are self-employed, you'll need to track your wages more closely and base your plan on your average monthly income.

Second, keep track of all of your spending and divide it up into the three categories of essentials, flexible spending, and financial goals. Now, if you're overspending in one of the categories, adjust it so you're falling into the 50/30/20 parameters.

For example, if you're making $3,000 a month, your budget should be $1,500 for essentials, $900 for flexible spending, and $600 for financial goals. If you're spending $2,000 on essentials, then you have to cut it by at least $500. The easiest way to do this is by cutting the big three: transportation, food, and housing. One suggestion is to add a roommate who pays $750 a month, this way you're covering the extra $500 you went over on your essentials category, and now you have an extra $250 to go into one of your other categories, like financial goals.

There are several ways to save on transportation, like carpooling, riding a bike, or using public transportation.

Food is tricky because you want to save on the sources of food but not on the quality. For example, a friend of mine and his wife really wanted to buy a nice house so they started eating top ramen every day for a year. They saved a lot of money and bought a house. But I don't believe that the collateral damage from the high salt and low nutrition was worth it, because they ended up with high blood pressure. Instead, keep eating high-quality organic fruits and veggies, and cut back on eating out and substitute with economical options.

Overall the strategy is to cut as much as you can from the essentials and flexible spending categories so you can add more to the financial goals category.

The 50-30-20 Rule works, because it's simple and everything is clearly defined, making it much more likely that you'll stick to your plan and meet your financial goals. It also allows you to adjust percentages to help you meet your goals faster.

For strategies on how to boost your income while not working and recovering from your injury check out; *How to Become Rich and Successful: Creative Ways to Make Money with a Side Hustle. How to Become a Millionaire - Learn the Best Passive Income Ideas.*

Chapter 28: How to Travel the World in a Wheelchair or on Crutches

Traveling requires special planning and preparation if you're in a wheelchair or on crutches. The complexity of your trip will grow depending on your level of disability. By understanding the variables that could slow your journey, you can plan accordingly to overcome them.

If you've recently had surgery, speak to your doctor regarding travel restrictions. Typically, after surgery, you're at higher risk for blood clots for up to six months, and plane travel increases the risk even more. When scheduling your flights, extend layovers between connecting flights to decrease the risk of blood clots. Keep in mind that the longer the trip, the higher the risk of blood clots.

If your mobility is limited or you've recently had surgery, make sure you are moving your body every 1-2 hours for a few minutes to reduce the risk of blood clots. If you're able to stand supported, do toe raises. If you can't stand, then move your limbs while seated and complete isometric exercises. For example, press your hands together in a prayer position as hard as you can for ten seconds. You'll feel the tension in your chest and arms, yet your arms didn't move at all. For your legs, push your feet into the ground as hard as you can for ten seconds, so you'll feel the tension in your feet and legs. These are isometric exercises where you have the static contraction of a muscle without any visible movement in the angle of the joint allowing your muscles to pump and circulate blood through the limb, which significantly reduces the risk of blood clots. Keep in mind to maintain your weight-bearing precautions if you have any. For example, if you're not supposed to put weight on your leg, don't stand on it; instead, use isometric exercises.

Before you start your trip, learn the rules so your trip will go smoother. The Americans with Disabilities Act covers people in the USA while on the ground, and the Air Carrier Access Act (ACAA) covers access on all flights to and from the US. Familiarizing yourself with the laws will help you understand what accommodations, facilities, and services should be available to you. It's a good idea to carry a copy with you in case you have issues with staff who may not be familiar with the accommodations they are required to provide according to the law. If you have access-related questions, you can call the disability hotline operated by the US Department of Transportation at (800) 778-4838. If you have any pre-trip questions regarding the security screening process, contact the TSA at least 72 hours before your flight at (855) 787-2227.

Once you arrive at the airport, if you can't walk through the metal detector unassisted, let the airport security or Transportation Security Administration (TSA) agent know. They will take you aside, hand-wand you, and give you a manual pat-down. Let the agents know if you have any sore or tender body parts before the screening. You also have the option for a private screening, if you prefer, with a companion of your choice present.

Wheelchair Accommodations

1. If you're not able to walk long distances, request an airport wheelchair when you make your reservation. If you plan on traveling with your wheelchair, let the airline know beforehand what type of an assistive device you have. Passengers with battery-powered wheelchairs have to arrive at the airport at least one hour before standard check-in time.

2. When making your plane reservations, request a seat with a flip-up armrest, which will make transfers much more manageable. A bulkhead is a divider that separates the classes or sections of a plane. These seats have extra legroom and are therefore easier to get in an out. Although not required by the ACAA, some airlines will routinely block bulkhead seats for passengers with limited mobility.

3. The ACAA also entitles you to stay in your wheelchair (if it has non-spillable batteries) until you get to the gate. Once you get to the gate, your wheelchair will be taken down to the cargo area, and you'll be transported to your seat in a high-back aisle chair if you can't walk. Once you get to your destination, your wheelchair or scooter will be delivered to you at the gate.

4. Bring assembly and disassembly instructions (in Spanish and English) for your mobility device with you to the airport. The ACAA requires that if a wheelchair or scooter is disassembled for transport, it must be returned to the passenger correctly assembled. Having assembly instructions available to the staff who'll be helping will make things easier.

5. Planes that have more than one hundred seats have storage space aboard for one manual wheelchair. This space is available on a first-come basis, so try to get to the boarding area early.

6. Before you board the plane use the airport bathrooms, since they tend to be easier to access. Airplane bathrooms are small, and you need to be able to walk a few steps to use them. So have a backup plan such as wearing a diaper, in case you have an accident, it'll be easier to clean up.

7. Remember, many people are on crutches or wheelchairs, and airline staff have their protocols for helping such passengers. Ask for priority boarding and request special services staff to assist you.

8. Book hotels, tours, and trips to places that are wheelchair accessible. Pre-planning is vital, so you don't end up somewhere where wheelchair accessibility is not a consideration. If the location is not accessible and you have the funds, you can make the place convenient for you by paying for private transportation and traveling with your wheelchair ramp, adaptive equipment, and a travel partner who can help you manage your equipment and help you access the location you're visiting. Check out *Curb Free with Cory Lee* for examples and strategies used by Cory Lee on how he travels the world in his power wheelchair.

Accommodations for Travelers with Crutches

If you're able to self-ambulate with crutches and partially weight bear, then you may be able to navigate most environments. However, airports may require long waits in lines for check-in or security clearance. Therefore, it's best to make arrangements with the airport before you arrive to have a wheelchair provided to you, to help you navigate the airport easier and decrease the risk of you falling due to fatigue.

1. Again you can request bulkhead seating. If you can afford the expense, upgrade to a higher-class seat, or ask to be seated next to empty seats, so you have more room to navigate. The same goes for wheelchairs users.

2. Hotels in developed countries have a limited number of accessible rooms available. So book rooms in advance so you can have a room with wider doorways and spacious bathrooms that make it easier for you to move around. Otherwise, most hotels have tub-shower combos, which are not accessible in a wheelchair and complicated when you're on crutches. Accessible rooms will usually provide a walk-in shower, grab bars, and a detachable showerhead.

3. Book hotels in advance and request rooms on the ground floor or near the elevator. If you'll need a wheelchair while on hotel grounds, reserve a wheelchair in advance with the hotel.

4. Make advanced preparations to see which airport shuttles and car rental buses can accommodate you. In developed countries, most transportation is fitted to support wheelchairs and folks with limited mobility on crutches.

5. Public transportation in developed countries typically have signs, symbols, and are wheelchair accessible.

6. Traveling will require you to expend more energy than you usually do in your everyday life. Therefore, it's best to train for your trip by spending more time walking on your crutches and/or wheeling yourself in your wheelchair.

7. If you can afford the expense, consider buying lighter mobility equipment for traveling. Items such as a lighter wheelchair, walker, lighter crutches, collapsible crutches, transport wheelchair, lighter cane, or a device that's easier to break down will make your trip easier.

8. Lighten your load as much as possible. Use luggage and materials that are lightweight, so you expend less energy moving your items. If possible, pack everything into one backpack, so it's less to keep track of and more comfortable for people who are helping you.

9. Keep in mind that you're going to need more time to navigate airports, hotels, and tourist sites, so schedule extra time for everything you do so you're not rushed and put yourself into danger trying to rush to places.

10. Keep vital travel documents where they are easily accessible in a fanny pack. Bring extra $1 bills so that you can tip the attendants and anyone who helps facilitate your journey.

11. Be cool; stress, pain, and discomfort can be magnified by the fatigue of traveling, so remember to stay calm and courteous to others.

If you run into access-related problems while at the airport, ask to speak to the Complaints Resolution Official (CRO); all airlines in the US are required to have a CRO on duty during airport operating hours. This airline employee is specially trained in the ACAA and can resolve access-related issues on the spot.

If the CRO is unable to assist you, file a written complaint with the airline after you return home. Sometimes this can be your best and only option for receiving monetary compensation for damages. Be mindful of deadlines, as airlines are not required to respond to complaints postmarked more than forty-five days after the incident. For complaints filed on time, the airlines must respond within thirty days.

If these two steps have not resolved your complaint,

then you can file a complaint with the DOT for access-related problems. Claims must be done within six months of the incident and can result in changes to airline policies and practices. Filing a complaint can help make air travel more accessible.

I was fortunate enough to have the opportunity to travel in a wheelchair and on crutches. Some of the critical issues that quickly became apparent to me:

1. Be patient, as many people mean well, but not everyone will be familiar with your needs and limitations. Also, keep in mind that most people are not patient, so they will avoid you or try not to help you, not always because they don't want to but because they are worried that they won't be able to provide the help you need. Accept help where you can, and when people can't or won't, don't stress about it. Move on to the next person, or take the time to educate the person on your needs and on how they can help you. Explain that even though you might not be able to do things the way others do, you can still enjoy being there and experiencing it your way.

2. Although I'm 6' 2", 210 lbs., and have years of experience in martial arts, I felt an immediate sense of vulnerability, and this is normal when you're in a wheelchair or on crutches. So avoid situations where others can take advantage of or cause your harm. I usually avoided exploring dark streets at night, brought a companion with me to dangerous countries, and used transportation to avoid moving through areas of higher risk. Don't allow fear to force you into staying home, most people are conscious of people with disabilities, and I've experienced extreme kindness from folks from all around the world. People who were helpful and went out of their way to assist me when no one required them to do so. Most people will respect and admire you for taking on the challenge and try to help; however, they can.

Nonetheless you must be aware of your limitations and avoid situations where you could be at a significant disadvantage. Try to join groups, inquire before and avoid dangerous areas; stay away from lonely or dimly lit places, don't accept private rides or tours from strangers. When you go out, inform the hotel staff of your plans and anticipated return times. I'd also recommend checking in with someone at home regularly so they are aware of where you are in case you need assistance.

3. Be conservative with your plans, and don't try to pack too many activities into one day. It's best to leave extra time for completing the activities, so you're not under time constraints, since you won't be able to complete them as you usually would. Most things are going to take longer than they usually do, because you're going to have to wait for elevators, assistance from staff, and you're going to need extra rest breaks.

4. Allow extra time for sleep and recovery. Typically, when I travel, I can withstand being on my feet for up to sixteen hours a day walking and sightseeing, but while in a wheelchair or on crutches, a few hours were often enough to leave me exhausted. Remember, your body is meant to move you around most efficiently while on two legs. If you're using your arms to propel a wheelchair, you have a battery-powered wheelchair, or have to use your shoulders and arms to move you around on a pair of crutches; you're going to be moving in a much less efficient manner than a person normally would, and you're going to be expending much more energy as well. Give yourself extra time to sleep and take breaks throughout the day, so you don't exert yourself too much and cause yourself to get tendonitis, strains, or muscle tears. As mentioned before, make sure you prepare for your trip by spending extra time mobilizing yourself and preparing your body for the extra endurance needed to travel.

5. Start with more comfortable travel destinations until you get up to speed. Being stuck inside for months on end can be boring and depressing, but I was unsure of how to proceed because I felt vulnerable. So, I started with road trips in the western USA with my cousin Miska. I was unable to drive because of all the hardware installed on my body, and I needed help unloading my wheelchair;

therefore, Miska drove, and I was the passenger. As my endurance and travel know-how increased, we went to first-world destinations like Hawaii. As my mobility improved, even more, I set out solo with crutches to countries such as Mexico, and I used a walking cane in the jungles of Suriname, Guyana, and French Guiana. As you experience early success in your travels, you will slowly work out the bugs, develop strategies, and gain confidence in how to do things.

6. Use social media to connect with other people with limited mobility, who live at the travel destinations you'd like to visit, and get ideas about strategies you can use to navigate the local environment.

7. Know that it is typical for a person with limited mobility to have to pay more for tours and other services. You are going to require more time and effort from the hosts, so don't be taken aback when you hear they may be charging you more than others. It's not personal; it's economics, so don't let that be a deterrent to engaging in activities. You never know when or if you'll have the opportunity to experience something special.

For more travel tips check out; *How to Travel the World and Live with No Regrets. Learn How to Travel for Free, Find Cheap Places to Travel, and Discover Life-Changing Travel Destinations.*

Conclusion

The bone is considered one of nature's marvels. Bones are the foundation for many living organisms and can last up to a few geologic eras. Of all the components of the human body, the bone is the most biologically diverse

You'll never be ready for a broken bone when it does happen, rest assured that your body is generally able to deal with it. However, if you're older, have an illness, had severe trauma, or simply want to get back on your feet quickly so you can get back to work or compete in your sport, this book will give you some ideas that you can share with your medical team to help you heal faster. Just keep in mind that although your situation may seem dire, people break bones all the time and they heal. Keep a positive outlook and stay focused on the end goal of getting back to your wonderful life.

About the Author

Dr. Ernesto Martinez suffered a near-fatal assault that changed the direction of his life. The experience helped him acquire a greater moral understanding and develop greater empathy for others.

Martinez is a Naturopathic Doctor, Occupational Therapist, and Investor. He also enjoys writing, publishing, traveling, blogging AttaBoyCowboy.com, and running his YouTube channel AttaBoyCowboy.

So be sure to check out his fun books, blog, and YouTube channel.

Martinez's work as a Naturopathic Doctor specializes in anti-aging medicine and complementary cancer therapies. He focuses on a whole-body treatment approach utilizing safe natural methods, while simultaneously restoring the body's natural ability to heal.

His work as an Occupational Therapist has allowed him to help people across the lifespan to do things they want and need to do to live their life to the fullest. His strong desire to mentor and help others has led him to teach, share, and help them live better lives.

As an Investor, Martinez has focused his training and business acumen on real estate. With a family history of real estate investing and extensive academic training, he has developed innovative strategies for building wealth from nothing.

In addition to his medical practice and three decades of investing experience, Martinez is making his impact on the writing and media field. Through his books, blog, and YouTube channel, he is reaching a broad spectrum of people and teaching them how to live healthier and wealthier lives.

Martinez has taught extension courses at the University of San Diego in topics ranging from nutrition and general health to leadership and business. He holds five associate degrees from Cerritos College, a bachelor's degree from the University of Southern California (USC), an MBA in economics and marketing, and a master's degree in healthcare management (MHCM) from California State University Los Angeles (CSULA), a doctoral degree from Clayton College, and over ten other degrees and advanced certifications in areas including lifestyle redesign and nutrition, alternative nutrition, assistive technology, sensory integration, neuro-developmental treatment, physical agent modalities, lymphedema treatment, and property management. He studied over fifteen years working his entire academic career and for several years attending two graduate schools on two separate campuses at the same time.

He is a huge fan of all sports, reading, and being on the road traveling!

As an entrepreneur, Ernesto is usually problem-solving business issues, writing, and learning to be a better person. He enjoys spending time with his family and friends.

By far one of his favorite activities is practicing his Random Acts of Kindness, where he tries to do three acts of kindness for strangers a day.

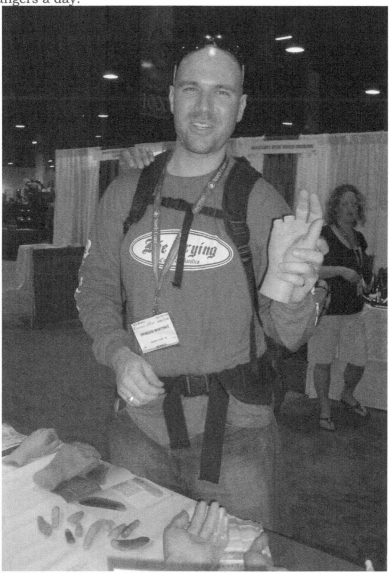

How to Heal Broken Bones Faster. Bone Fracture Healing Tips.

Bonus

Top Ten Ways to Decrease Your Environmental Impact During Travel per World Wildlife Fund (WWF)

1. Go on holiday during the off-peak period to prevent overstraining resources; you'll also avoid the crowds.

2. Find out about places before you visit. You may be visiting an environmentally sensitive area, in which case you must take extra care to stay on footpaths and follow signs.

3. Don't travel by air if you can avoid it, because air travel uses up large amounts of jet fuel that releases greenhouse gases.

4. Dispose of any rubbish responsibly; it can be hazardous to wildlife.

5. Use public transportation, cycle or walk instead of using a car.

6. Use facilities and trips run by local people whenever possible.

7. Don't be tempted to touch wildlife and disturb habitats whether on land, at the coast, or under water.

8. Be careful what you choose to bring home as a holiday souvenir. Many species from coral and conch shells to elephants and alligators are endangered because they are killed for curios or souvenirs.

9. Don't dump chemicals into the environment; it can be very dangerous for wildlife.

10. Boats and jet-skis create noise and chemical pollution that is very disturbing to wildlife; don't keep the engine running unnecessarily

Top Ten Ways to Decrease Your Environmental Impact

after Travel per WWF

1. Completely turn off equipment like televisions and stereos when you're not using them.

2. Choose energy-efficient appliances and light bulbs.

3. Save water: some simple steps can go a long way in saving water, like turning off the tap when you are brushing your teeth or shaving. Try to collect the water used to wash vegetables and salad to water your houseplants.

4. Lower your shades or close your curtains on hot days, to keep the house fresh and reduce the use of electric fans or air-conditioning.

5. Let clothes dry naturally.

6. Keep lids on pans when cooking to conserve energy.

7. Use rechargeable batteries.

8. Call your local government to see if they have a disposal location for used batteries, glass, plastics, paper, or other wastes.

9. Don't use "throwaway" products like paper plates and napkins or plastic knives, forks, and cups.

10. Send electronic greetings over email instead of paper cards.

Top Ten Ways to Decrease Your Environmental Impact in the Garden per WWF

1. Collect rainwater to water your garden.

2. Water the garden early in the morning or late in the evening. Water loss is reduced due to evaporation. Don't over-water the garden. Water only until the soil becomes moist, not soggy.

3. Explore water-efficient irrigation systems. Sprinkler irrigation and drip irrigation can be adapted to garden situations.

4. Make your garden lively, plant trees, and shrubs that will attract birds. You can also put up bird nest boxes with food.

5. Put waste to work in your garden, sweep the fallen leaves and flowers into flowerbeds, or under shrubs. Increasing soil fertility and also reduce the need for frequent watering.

6. If you have little space in your garden, you could make a compost pit to turn organic waste from the kitchen and garden to soil-enriching manure.

7. Plant local species of trees, flowers, and vegetables.

8. Don't use chemicals in the garden, as they will eventually end up in the water systems and can upset the delicate balance of life cycles.

9. Organic and environmentally friendly fertilizers and pesticides are available - organic gardening reduces pollution and is better for wildlife.

10. Buy fruit and vegetables that are in season to help reduce enormous transport costs resulting from importing products and, where possible, choose locally produced food.

Top Ten Ways to Reduce, Reuse, and Recycle per WWF

1. Use email to stay in touch, including cards, rather than faxing or writing.

2. Share magazines with friends and pass them on to the doctor, dentist, or local hospital for their waiting rooms.

3. Use recyclable paper to make invitation cards,

envelopes, letter pads, etc. if you can.

4. Use washable nappies instead of disposables, if you can.

5. Recycle as much as you can.

6. Give unwanted clothes, toys, and books to charities and orphanages.

7. Store food and other products in containers rather than foil and plastic wrap.

8. When buying fish, look out for a variety of non-endangered species, and buy local fish if possible.

9. Bring your bags to the grocery and refuse plastic bags that create so much waste.

10. Look for products that have less packaging.

Top Ten Ways to Reduce Your Environmental Impact at Work per WWF

1. Always use both sides of a sheet of paper.

2. Use printers that can print on both sides of the paper; try to look into this option when replacing old printers.

3. Use the back of a draft or unwanted printout instead of notebooks. Even with a double-sided printer, there is likely to be plenty of spare paper to use!

4. Always ask for and buy recycled paper if you can, for your business stationery, and to use it in your printers.

5. Switch off computer monitors, printers, and other equipment at the end of each day. Always turn off your office light and computer monitor when you go out for lunch or to a meeting.

6. Look for power-saving alternatives like LED light bulbs, motion-sensing to control the lighting, LED computer monitors, etc. Prioritize buying or replacing equipment and appliances with their higher Energy Rating alternatives.

7. Contact your energy provider and what they offer in the way of green energy alternatives. You could install solar panels to reduce reliance on energy providers if they're slow on the green energy uptake.

8. Carpool. Ask your workmates that live nearby if they'd be happy to share rides with you.

9. Be smarter with your company vehicles. When reviewing your fleet, spend some time researching more efficient cars.

10. Clean and maintain equipment regularly to extend their useful life and avoid having to replace them. Just like getting your vehicle serviced regularly, your floors, kitchens, equipment, and bathrooms all need regular attention to protect their form and function.

Made in the USA
Las Vegas, NV
23 August 2024

94271627R00135